Greek Medical Manuscripts
Diels' Catalogue

Tome 4: Ceteri Medici

Medical Traditions

Edited by
Alain Touwaide

Volume 2/4

De Gruyter

Greek Medical Manuscripts
Diels' Catalogue

Tome 4: Ceteri Medici

Newly revised and updated by
Alain Touwaide

De Gruyter

ISBN 978-3-11-060069-8
e-ISBN (PDF) 978-3-11-060199-2
ISSN 2567-6938

Library of Congress Control Number: 2020945916

Bibliographic information published by the Deutsche Nationalbibliothek
The Deutsche Nationalbibliothek lists this publication in the Deutsche Nationalbibliografie; detailed bibliographic data are available on the Internet at http://dnb.dnb.de.

Printing: CPI books GmbH, Leck
Cover image: Collage of illustrations in medical treatises from the 1st to the 16th century CE, from Greece and Rome, to the Arabic World and China.

www.degruyter.com

Table of contents

Foreword

The study of Greek manuscripts of medical content has seen a significant, though not exclusive, investigation by Alain Touwaide, whose life of scholar has been entirely devoted to the knowledge and valorization of the medical traditions of the Mediterranean world with a particular reference to the history of ancient and medieval Greek medicine.

The revisions and updates of the catalogues of Greek medical manuscripts compiled in the early 20th century by an équipe of philologists, guided by the distinguished historian of ancient Greek philosophy and medicine Hermann Diels (*Die Handschriften der antiken Ärzte*), are a cornerstone of Touwaide's scientific research on medical manuscripts, the further developments of which already include plans for a detailed catalogue of all surviving witnesses according to the norms of modern catalography.

Four years after his 2016 voluminous *Census of Greek Medical Manuscripts*, the publication of this new and substantial reference work constitutes a further step, complementary to the previous one, of his programme that will ultimately allow for the critical edition of a series of Greek medical texts in a way reminiscent of the *Corpus Medicorum* conceived by Diels over a century ago as the natural outcome of the catalogues of manuscripts that he coordinated.

If Alain Touwaide embarked on an arduous task with his *Census* and the compilation of an updated list of Greek manuscripts with medical contents—many of which were not listed in Diels' early 20th-century catalogues—the completion of a renewed Diels is a no less demanding endeavour. Diels' catalogues, which have been the reference for over a century for any scholar interested in the study of late antique and medieval Greek medicine from any perspective, are known, indeed, to suffer several limitations—besides the incompleteness of their inventory of manuscripts (well highlighted by the numerous complements provided in the *Census*)—that can be traced to the difficulty in identifying manuscripts generated by Diels' use of shelfmarks which have been made obsolete since by changes in the name of libraries or collections, in ownership, or in the location of collections. To further make research laborious, the printing of Diels' original edition is rather unclear.

Alain Touwaide has chosen to exactly reproduce the substance of Diels' work, even though he significantly intervened with great acumen on the structure, citation format, and presentation of the text, to make its contents more immediately usable and its consultation easier. An innovative organization of data in five tomes (in which the reproduction of Diels' original text in a decidedly more readable form is followed by two different methods of accessing the information, by type of contents—in tomes two through four—and by manuscript—in the fifth and final tome) is accompanied by an articulated system of indices designed to combine the need to reproduce Diels' original text *ad litteram* and the scientific imperative to update and standardize the method of referencing the manuscripts, and also to multiply the keys for searching the texts. In this view, Touwaide's decision to split the list of authors and works is revealing as it allows for the identification of texts by both their Greek and Latin title (albeit following the form, which is not always consistent, of the titles in Diels' original version), thus providing a first effort for a future standardization. Equally inspired by a justifiable need for clarity and simplification is the choice of accompanying the index of the original shelfmarks of manuscripts with a list of the English names of the cities and libraries. Finally, the layout of this renewed Diels clearly improves on the original edition, structuring its presentation in a much clearer and more effective way through different levels of indentation.

Those who are acquainted with Alain Touwaide know that only his visionary and tenacious spirit, supported by an unshakable patience and a truly extraordinary work capacity, could have pushed him to embark alone on the revision of the catalogues that Diels conceived and could complete thanks to the collaboration of a team of no fewer than thirty scholars. Touwaide's revision required many long years of meticulous work, with a sheer quantity of doublechecks, corrections, and identifications of new locations and shelfmarks, as well as *in situ* autoptic inspection of many manuscripts and sometimes even of entire collections.

Though constantly making explicit its connection with Diels' original work through its coherent and functional system of cross-references, the present revision of Diels will ultimately make it unnecessary to refer to the old Diels and make it possible, instead, to work only with updated lists of manuscripts. Furthermore, the multiple indices extremely well designed by Touwaide and the cross-referencing they make possible pave the way to a future, highly desirable transfer of data from a printed form to an open database, much of the necessary material of which is contained in the present work, in addition to the new data already provided by the *Census*. It can be expected that such a database will be constantly expanded and updated by integrating the results of the new developments and research that the catalogue that we have here will undoubtedly contribute to, promote, and generate.

The renewed Diels that we have here deserves to be hailed as an invaluable reference for both the niche of scholars scrutinizing Greek medical manuscripts and texts, and the wider circle of the historians of medicine, pharmacy, and ancient and medieval science, in a way that faithfully reflects the cross-disciplinary approach to the study of medical traditions that Alain Touwaide has convincingly advocated for for years in the name of a fruitful alliance of sciences and the humanities.

We now wish that, as a further contribution to the knowledge of the ancient Greek medical tradition, he will publish a much needed catalogue of Greek medical manuscripts and texts, not only those listed in Diels, but also the many new ones of which he has revealed the existence thanks to his unwavering energy, his devotion to research, and the passion for Greek medicine that has constantly distinguished his life.

Marilena Maniaci
Università degli Studi di Cassino e del Lazio meridionale
Rome, August 2, 2020

Introduction

Just over a century has passed since a team of scholars from across Europe, led by German historian of ancient philosophy and science Hermann Diels (1848–1922)[1], compiled the manuscripts containing Greek medical texts and their medieval translations into a catalogue[2]. Following such classical bibliographies as the *Bibliotheca Graeca* by Johann Albert Fabricius (1668–1736)[3] and the several *Bibliothecae* by Albrecht von Haller (1708–1777)[4], *Diels*, as the catalogue became known, was a landmark in classical and medico-historical scholarship[5]. It was not completely

---

1 For a broad approach to Diels' multifaceted activity, see for example Calder et al. 1999. All works referred to in this introduction are cited in an abbreviated form (author's last name and year of publication). For the full reference, see the bibliography at pp. xxi–xxx.

2 The catalogue was published in two issues in 1905 and 1906, in the proceedings of Berlin Academy of Science, with a supplement in 1908 in the same series (Diels 1905, 1906a, and 1908, respectively). The 1905 and 1906 issues were published together as a volume in 1906 (Diels 1906b) with a slightly different title (*Die Handschriften der antiken Ärzte, Griechische Abteilung*) which implied that a similar programme would have dealt with the Latin manuscripts. The frontmatter of the second issue (1906a), which provided a general presentation of the programme, the list of the collaborators, and the bibliography, is reproduced as the front matter of this volume with the same pagination as in the first publication. All three issues (1905, 1906a, and 1908) were reprinted in 1970 with an introduction by Fridolf Kudlien (1928–2008) (Kudlien 1970). The translations under consideration were those in Syriac, Arabic, Hebrew, and Latin according to the treatises.
All references to the catalogue here and in the present work comprise two elements: the first identifies the issue of the catalogue (I, II, or N [for *Nachtrag* = Supplement]), and the second (in Arabic numerals) provides the number of the page(s) referred to (e.g., I.22 or N.49). A number in Arabic numerals between parentheses after the second element, such as e.g., II.63 (2), indicates the number of mentions of a manuscript on the same page.

3 Fabricius' *Bibliotheca Graeca* was originally published in 14 volumes between 1705 and 1728, with a second edition started as early as 1708 and pursued until 1754, and also a third edition of Volumes 1 and 2 published in 1718 and 1752, respectively. The whole *Bibliotheca* was further published in a revised edition by Gottlieb Christopher Harles (1738–1815) in 12 volumes published between 1790 and 1809, with an *Index* in 1838. Under the general designation *Bibliotheca Graeca*, all volumes have a distinctive title that indicates their respective contents. In the first volume this title makes an explicit reference to manuscripts (... *notitia Scriptorum Veterum Graecorum quorumcunque monumenta integra, aut fragmenta edita exstant: tum plerorumque è MSS. ac deperditis* ...). On Fabricius, see Verner 1966.

4 The first of Haller's *Bibliothecae* was the *Bibliotheca botanica* (1771–1772), which included large chapters on ancient physicians (see for example, Dioscorides, vol. 1, pp. 79–87 [page 79 is numbered 97]). It was followed by the *Bibliotheca chirurgica* (1774–1775), the *Bibliotheca anatomica* (1774–1777), and the *Bibliotheca medicinae practicae* (1776–1788).

5 For the history of the search for the manuscripts of Greek medical texts from the Renaissance to Diels, see Touwaide 2009, particularly pp. 456–508.

unprecedented, however. From the late eighteenth century on, several similar compilations were made, indeed, but they relied either on earlier literature or on *in situ* inspection of just some collections by single scholars. These were the bibliographies compiled by Johann Christian Gottlieb Ackermann (1756–1801)[6] and the pioneering search for manuscripts by the German scholar Friedrich Reinhold Dietz (1804–1836) in the 1830s[7], followed shortly after by the exploratory missions of the French historian of medicine Charles Daremberg (1817–1872), mostly in England[8], with a similar collection of material *in loco* at the Bibliothèque nationale in Paris by the Greek ophthalmologist Georges Costomiris (1849–1902)[9]. Diels' enterprise was different in its systematicity and scale, in addition to its organization, its team[10], and its international network[11] which combined in-house bibliographical research[12] and *in-*

6 Ackermann's bibliographies with their lists of manuscripts for Hippocrates, Dioscorides and Galen, were published in Harles' edition of Fabricius' *Bibliotheca Graeca* (vol. 2 [1791], pp. 506–611, 4 [1795], pp. 673–702, and 5 [1796], pp. 377–500, respectively). The lists of Hippocratic and Galenic manuscripts were reproduced in the edition of these authors in Kühn's *Medicorum Graecorum Opera quae exstant* under the title *Historia literaria* (for Hippocrates, see vol. 1 [1825], pp. I–CCVI; for Galen, see vol. 1 [1821]), pp. XIX–CCLXV). Interestingly enough, Diels referred to these two lists. The list of manuscripts for Dioscorides, *De materia medica*, in Kühn's *Medicorum Graecorum Opera quae exstant* (see vol. 1 [1829], pp. XX–XXVI) did not reproduce Ackermann's, but was compiled by the editor of the text, Kurt Sprengel (1766–1833).

7 Dietz traveled through Germany, Italy, Spain, France, and Britain, systematically searching for codices containing Greek medical texts (see Dietz 1832: IX–X; Dietz 1834: 1.IV), principally Hippocrates, but also Oribasius (he was supposed to prepare an edition for the corpus edited by Kühn), Aetius, the commentators on Hippocrates, Ioannes Zacharias Actuarius, Greek chemical works, Soranus, Paul of Aegina, Rufus of Ephesus, Erotianus, Nicander, Theophilus, Symeon Seth, and others (e.g., Severus iatrosophist whose treatise he published [Dietz 1836]).

8 See the reports of his travels in Daremberg 1845, 1848, 1851, and 1852, with a reproduction of the last two in the form of a monograph in 1853.

9 Costomiris published the results of his investigations at the Bibliothèque nationale in a series of five contributions to the *Revue des études grecques* published between 1889 and 1897.

10 The collaborators of the program are listed in the front matter of the 1906 issue and the 1906 reprint (p. X) with some further names in the 1908 supplement (p. 23). Besides the collaborators *in loco* (among whom were Ph.D. candidates) coordinated in collaboration by Diels and Johan Ludwig Heiberg (1854–1928), the team included several German scholars as Joseph Heeg (1881–1916) in Munich, Georg Helmreich (1849–1921) in Ansbach, Johannes Ilberg (1860–1930) in Leipzig, Karl Kalbfleich (1868–1946) in Marburg, Iwan von Müller (1830–1917) at that time in Munich, Paul Schwarz (1867–1938), then in Berlin, and Max Wellmann (1863–1933). Their number was higher, however, as the reading of the catalogues indicates: the annotations that accompany the mention of some manuscripts refer to scholars whose name does not appear in the two lists of collaborators.

11 The list of collaborators includes several individuals from abroad who were librarians or academics with a special interest in the history of ancient medicine and medical literature, including translations. These scholars were the following (in alphabetical order of last name): Hartwig (Henry) Derembourg (1844–1908) in Paris; Eduard Gottlob (1856–1922) in Krems a.

situ examination of entire library collections by local scholars or members of Diels' team in mission abroad[13].

Remarkably enough, the vast collection of data contained in the two issues of Diels' catalogues was assembled in barely four years[14], witnessing an exceptional mobilization of efforts and resources[15]. Although a supplement—presented as the first—was published in 1908, it was not followed by any other. Shortly after, the team lost some of its collaborators in the First World War[16], and the systematic search for the manuscripts of ancient medical texts was no longer pursued. Nevertheless, several

---

d. Donau; Montague Rhodes James (1862–1936) in Cambridge; Philip Christian Molhuysen (1870–1944) in Leiden; Alessandro Olivieri (1872–1950) in Naples; Adriano Piccolomini (1843–1907) in Cesena; Anton Ritter von Premerstein (1869–1935) in Vienna; Hans Raeder (1859–1969) in Copenhagen; Walter Scott (1855–1925) in Oxford, with a parenthesis in Montreal (1905–1908); Hermann Schöne (1870–1941) in Basel; Rezső Vári (1867–1940) in Budapest, and Eric Otto Windstedt (1880–1955) in Oxford. This list is not exhaustive, however, as other names appear scattered in the catalogues. The different collaborators interacted as the references to collations (see below) indicate.

12 The consulted bibliography (listed in the 1906a issue [pp. XI–XXIII] with a supplement in 1908 [pp. 23–24]) does not account for the full extent of the library resources consulted by the collaborators of the catalogues, which contain scattered references to works not included in the bibliographical lists.

13 One such mission was that of Max Wellmann, who spent 1906–1907 in Italy, where he particularly investigated the collections of the Vatican and the Marciana libraries. As a result, the 1908 supplement contains multiple annotations made on the basis of his personal consultation of manuscripts.

14 To give an idea of the sheer quantity of data presented in the catalogues, suffice it to say that the number of items from Greek manuscripts only amounts to over 14,000. To this we should add the multiple collations of manuscripts made by the collaborators of the programme during *in loco* research stays or on their behalf that are mentioned in the catalogue. Ilberg, for example, collated himself or received collations of most of the Hippocratic writings from manuscripts at the Vatican Library, and in Florence, Venice, Vienna, and Paris, whereas Helmreich concentrated on Galen (in one case at least, he had a collation of all but one manuscript of a Galenic treatise; see I.83–84).

15 For the history of the programme, see Kollesch 1973, 1989, and 1999; and more recently, Nutton 2004.

16 This was the case of Bruno Rappaport (1875–1915), who managed the data of the catalogues in collaboration with Joahnnes Mewald (1880–1964). On this, see Diels' introductory remarks (*Vorbemerkungen*) to the catalogue (Diels 1906a: pp. I–IX), which include the reports by Rappaport (pp. III–VI) and Mewaldt (pp. VI–VIII). On Rappaport, see the obituary by Regling, 1920. Another victim of the First World War was Joseph Heeg. During the compilation of the catalogues, the program lost another of its members, the orientalist Ludwig Nix (1865–1904) who had collected much material about the Arabic translations of Greek medical works.

editions of Greek medical texts were published thanks to the material collected during the compiling of the catalogues[17].

Addenda and *corrigenda* to Diels[18], studies of the manuscripts or tradition of specific medical treatises[19], and the systematic inventory of the manuscripts of texts to be edited, with the analysis of their tradition[20], punctuated the twentieth-century scholarship devoted to the ancient medical literature. After World War II, an

17 The first such edition was that of Philumenus, *De venenatis animalibus*, by Max Wellmann who discovered the text in the manuscript *Vaticanus graecus* 284 during his research stay at the Vatican Library (Wellmann 1908). This edition, which inaugurated the *Corpus Medicorum Graecorum*, brilliantly illustrated the function of the catalogues as a source of firsthand material for the preparation of the critical editions to be published in the *Corpus*. It is probably significant that it was followed in 1914 by the edition of the Arabic translation of a Pseudo-Galenic treatise by Gotthelf Bergsträsser (1886–1933) (Bergsträsser 1914), and the first edition of Galen in the *Corpus* by three collaborators of the programme (Mewaldt et al. 1914). Another Galenic edition, prepared by another group of three collaborators, followed the next year (Diels et al. 1915), together with Celsus by Friedrich Marx (1869–1941) and, the following year, Quintus Serenus Sammonicus by Friedrich Vollmer (1867–1923). After a short interruption due to World War I, no fewer than 15 editions were published between 1921 and 1937, with one edition every year from 1926 on, including (in chronological order of publication) the vast medical encyclopedias of Paul of Aegina (Heiberg 1921–1924), Oribasius (Raeder 1926, and 1928–1933), and Aetius (*partim*; Olivieri, 1935), in addition to the first Hippocratic edition (Heiberg et al., 1927), Soranus (Ilberg, 1927), Galenic commentaries on Hippocratic treatises (Wenkebach 1934 and 1936) and Galenic works (Koch et al. 1923; De Boer 1937). All this attested to the vitality of the *Corpus* and the usefulness of the catalogue.

18 As early as 1916, Giovanni Mercati (1866–1957), then a *scrittore* at the Vatican Library, published some *addenda* (Mercati 1916, 1917a, and 1917b). Corrections like these are scattered throughout twentieth-century scholarly publications related to the Greek medical literature. Most of them can be found in Touwaide 2016, *passim*, together with new ones. Additions and corrections to Diels' lists of manuscripts of the Latin translations of Greek medical texts have been systematically made, though later. Richard Durling (1932–1999) revised Diels' lists of the Galenic Latin manuscripts (Durling 1967 and 1981, completed only recently by Fortuna and Raia 2006; a cumulative catalogue of the Galenic and Pseudo-Galenic Latin texts [including manuscripts] compiled by Stefania Fortuna and her group is now available online in the form of a constant work in progress [*Galeno. Catalogo delle traduzioni latine*]). Pearl Kibre (1902–1985) compiled new lists of the Hippocratic Latin manuscripts in several installments (1975–1982) followed by a publication in the form of a monographic catalogue in 1985. It may be relevant to note here that Durling expanded his search for Latin medical manuscripts by browsing a collection of material similar to Diels, Kristeller's *Iter Italicum* (Durling 1985–1993).

19 An early work of this type is Ilberg 1911 on Soranus, followed shortly after by Diels 1912 on Galen's commentary on Hippocrates *Prorrheticum*, and Helmreich 1913 on Symeon Seth.

20 The best examples are the introductions to the editions published in the *Corpus Medicorum Graecorum* (which became more developed over time). Their template includes a list of manuscripts, their description, and a detailed philological analysis. Although these introductions focus on identifying the manuscript(s) to be used as a source or sources of the editions, they provide relevant data on codicology and book history.

unprecedented increase in the interest in paleography and codicology[21] soon led to a renewed search for, and study of, manuscripts[22], new catalogues[23], and, more recently, computerized databases allowing for the storage and multi-criteria querying of increasingly larger amounts of information[24], in addition to the digitization of the collections of manuscripts of several libraries across the world[25]. In the field of Greek medical manuscripts and texts, this resulted in the rediscovery or, in some cases, in the true discovery of manuscripts[26], new catalogues of medical manuscripts[27], the history

21 In the field of Greek codicology and palaeography, and also textual history, this interest was pioneered by such scholars as Joseph Mogenet (1913–1980), Herbert Hunger (1914–2000), Jean Irigoin (1920–2006), and Paul Canart (1927–2017). It subsequently led to an increased institutionalization of these disciplines illustrated, among others, by a series of international conferences started in 1974 (see *Paléographie,* 1977). For a recent esquisse of the history of codicology and paleography during the twentieth century, see, for example, Touwaide 2010.

22 Whereas the type of research by Alphonse Dain (1896–1964), Paul Henry (1906–1984), Alexander Turyn (1900–1981), and Jean Irigoin on technical texts (Dain 1930, 1933, 1946), Plotin (Henry 1938, 1941), the Greek tragics (Turyn 1943, 1952, 1957) and Pindar (Turyn 1932, and Irigoin 1952), respectively, was relatively rare until then in the academic production, it became more common later. For examples of such a line of investigation, see Eleuteri 1981 on a literary text (Musaeus) and Sonderkamp 1987 on a Greek medical treatise (Theophanes Nonnos/Chrysobalantes).

23 The increase in the publication of catalogues of manuscripts can be best measured by comparing the successive editions of the so-called *Richard* (Richard 1948, 1958, and 1964, followed by such a punctual review of new catalogues as Irigoin 1970, and the major updated editions of *Richard* by Olivier 1995 and 2018).

24 One such database is PINAKES currently hosted and maintained by the Section Grecque of the Institut de Recherche et d'Histoire des Textes (IRHT) of the Centre National de la Recherche Scientifique (CNRS), in Paris. It is built on the basis of the earlier research conducted at the Pontifical Institute of Medieval Studies at University of Toronto by Robert E. Sinkewicz, who compiled available printed catalogues of manuscripts and published the resulting data in the form of microfiches (Sinkewicz and Hayes 1989; Sinkewicz 1990 and 1992). In the matter of medical manuscripts and texts, see the database built on Diels accessible online through the website of the Institute for the Preservation of Medical Traditions. A precursor of this type of database was the catalogue of incipits of Latin medical treatises compiled as early as 1937 by Lynn Thorndike (1882–1965) and Pearl Kibre (1937). After a revised edition published in 1963, this catalogue has been complemented by Linda E. Voigts and Patricia D. Kurtz (Voigts and Kurz 2004), and transformed in digital form (first as a CD-Rom and now as a database consultable online on the site of the University of Missouri Kansas City).

25 See, for example, the site *Gallica*, of the Bibliothèque nationale de France, *teca* of the Biblioteca Medicea Laurenziana in Firenze, *DVL-DigiVatLib* of the Vatican Library, *DigitalBodleian*, *Digitised Manuscripts* of the British Library or, to mention just some, *e-codices* for the manuscripts in Swiss collections. Significantly enough, the most recent release of the site of the *Corpus Medicorum Graecorum* includes links to the digital version of the manuscripts of the authors for which critical editions have been published in the *Corpus*.

26 The most spectacular case has been the discovery of the forgotten manuscript Thessaloniki, Vlatadon 14, which contains a Galenic text which had remained unknown thus far. See Pietrobelli, 2010, for example. For other cases, see, for example, Roselli 2009 ([Hippocrates]) or

of collections of such codices[28], an accrued attention to medical illustration[29], studies of the textual tradition of Greek medical texts[30] or genres[31], the medical production of some regions[32], and new critical editions, particularly from the mid-twentieth century onward[33]. This activity, which also generated a forum in the form of a series of conferences launched by Antonio Garzya (1927–2012) in 1990 and regularly held

Perilli 2011 (Galen's Hippocratic lexicon), and Chatzopoulou 2014 and Tselikas 2014 about *iatrosofia*.

27 For some catalogues, see Hunger and Kresten as early as 1969 about the series *medici graeci* of the National Library of Austria in Vienna, and, more recently, Bouras-Vallianatos 2015 about the holdings of the Wellcome Library in London, with a short supplement in Bouras-Vallianatos 2020. A different type of catalogue is that of Formentin 1978, about the libraries of a region.

28 See, for example, Formentin 1997 about the medical manuscripts in the collection of the national library in Naples.

29 A pioneering work in this field was MacKinney 1965, which lists the medieval manuscripts known at that time in several languages with medical illustrations, with some descriptive elements. Recently see Bernabò 2010.

30 For the entire tradition of some works, see, for example (in chronological order of publication), Kudlien 1960 (Hippocrates, *De articulis*), Rivier 1962 (Hippocrates, *De morbo sacro*), and Alexanderson 1963 (Hippocrates, *Prognosticon*) and 1967 (Galen, *De crisibus*). Among the studies in subsequent years, one might cite Morani 1981 (Nemesius) or, more recently, Perilli 1999 (Galen's Hippocratic lexicon). Similar work is being done in Latin, for example by Green 1996 and 1997, on *Trotula*. Research was also devoted to some lesser-known physicians such as Mercurius (see the study by Masullo 2006), or to some segments or manuscripts of the tradition of one or more works. This is the case of Wilson 1987, for example, regarding a group of Galenic manuscripts (the codices copied by Ioannikios), and Petit 2006 on a group of manuscripts in relation with a text ([Galen], *Introductio*).

31 For this type of catalogue, see, for example, Ihm 2002 on medical commentaries (with references to the manuscripts), or Karas 1994, and Tselikas 1995 on *iatrosophia* (Byzantine and later).

32 For Southern Italy, for example, see Ieraci Bio 1989.

33 After an interruption provoked by World War II, the *Corpus Medicorum Graecorum* published anew critical editions as early as 1950 with a predilection for Galen, also including, however, Hippocratic treatises, Aretaeus, Rufus of Ephesus, Aetius, and Leo medicus, and, more recently (from 1983 on), Stephanus of Athens and Johannes of Alexandria. In the 1960s, the French *Collection des universités de France* launched a new Hippocrates (see Joly 1978 for the first volume; the programme has been pursued by Jacques Jouanna) and, very recently, a new Galen (see Boudon 2000 for the first volume). All this in addition to editions in series specifically devoted to the history of ancient and medieval/Byzantine medicine as *Studies in Ancient Medicine* (for example, Dickson 1998 on Stephanus, and Zipser 2009 on Johannes archiater) or, more recently, *Medicine in the Medieval Mediterranean* (Bennett 2016 on hospital formularies) and *Textos Médicos – Ediciones Críticas* (Lamagna 2017 on Johannes Actuarius' Greek translation of Avicenna, *De urinis*). See also such volumes as Pritchet 1975 and 1982 (both on Johannes of Alexandria) or Garzya and Masullo 2004 (on Cassius Iatrosophista). To this, one might add editions of *iatrosofia* (for example, Tselikas and Ilioudis 1995 and 1997, or Clark 2011).

since[34], was accompanied by a transformation in the history of science and the history of the book. While the former moved its focus from the *Great Scientists*[35] to the *histoire vécue*[36], the latter shifted from book production[37] to book use, that is, to reading, studying, annotating, sharing, and collecting[38].

Both transformational trends highlighted limitations of Diels' catalogues: they are devoted to authored works with a focus on the major physicians of classical antiquity and of the period that became defined in the meantime as *Late Antiquity*, that is, the period up to the end of the School of Alexandria in the 7th century A.D[39]. With only some exceptions[40], they omit the multiple small, but no less important, anonymous works, notebooks, and other formularies that give witness to the practice of medicine[41], and also many of the physicians of all epochs (but especially the Byzantine ones, also with some exceptions, however[42]) who have not been credited with such a foundational role as Hippocrates and Galen.

34 For the proceedings of the first conference, see Garzya 1992. The conference has been fairly consistently held every four years, alternately in Naples and Paris. The many communications presented in each edition dealt with a great many authors and texts, including lesser known physicians and their treatises. The proceedings were first edited by Antonio Garzya, and then by Garzya in collaboration with Jacques Jouanna before being edited by both, along with Véronique Boudon-Millot and Amneris Roselli.

35 As an example of this historiography, see the monumental encyclopedic *Introduction to the History of Science* (1927–1948) of George Sarton (1884–1956).

36 See, for example, Perrin 1988 on the skin (followed by Herida 1998, on skin in the Hippocratic writings), Rey 1993 on pain, or Dumouchel 1995 on emotions. One might also mention here the development of the history of the body, particularly its specific perception and its representation, including its defects (Fischer 1991).

37 The focus on book production might be best identified by the development of codicology, explicitly formalized as a discipline in its own right during this period (see Dain 1949).

38 On this approach, see, for example, the works of Guglielmo Cavallo, particularly Cavallo 1988 about libraries, and Cavallo and Chartier 1995 on reading, with a panoramic presentation of medieval reading culture. On reading Greek medical literature, more specifically, see, for example, Cavallo 1993 or, more recently, Mondrain 2003.

39 On the chonological span of the catalogues (from the 5th century B.C. to the 7th A.D.), see Bruno Rappaport's report in the 1906 issue, p. III.

40 Some of these exceptions might be the *Excerpta* (or *Excerpta varia*) listed for several authors, as well as the pseudepigraphic literature (mostly Hippocratic and Galenic) (see for example the remedies attributed to, or extracted from the works of, Hippocrates [I.48–49] and Galen [I.132–133]), in addition to some *iatrosophia* of the Ottoman period listed mostly under Hippocrates (I.42), Galen (I.123 and N.38) and Meletius (II.64), but also under Erasistratos (II.36) and Magnus (II.59), besides references to *iatrosophic* literature about Iustus (N.56), Logadius (N.56), Lucas (N.56), and Syncellus (N.66).

41 For such works (hospital formularies), see, for example, Bennett, 2016.

42 These exceptions are the following (in alphabetical order of their names as in Diels) with their reference to Diels: Abraham (II.3; N.42), Antonius Pyropulus (II.15; N.45), Beniaminus (II.22;

A *New Diels* is now a desideratum of the scholarly community[43]. While urgently needed, it would require that Greek medical manuscripts be newly catalogued and their texts accurately identified, building on the twentieth-century classical scholarship briefly presented above and indeed, going even further through a renewed *in situ* autoptic analysis of manuscripts and the reading of their many texts[44]. Whereas codicological analysis would allow for a better approximation of the time or period and place of production of the manuscripts (and also of their texts in some cases), reading and precise identification of all their texts would lead to a more complete and accurate knowledge of medical literature and practice from antiquity to the Renaissance, particularly thanks to the treatises of the period posterior to the 7th century and, for all periods, the multiple anonymous texts of all types not considered in Diels' catalogues.

The present work aims to lead the study of Greek medical manuscripts and literature of the classical and post-classical periods in that direction. While it fundamentally reproduces Diels' lists of Greek manuscripts, it reformats them in different, yet complementary, ways and provides new search tools that may be used for at least two purposes: compiling a catalogue of Greek medical manuscripts that will eventually generate the material necessary for a *New Diels*, and investigating the tradition, reception, and intellectual, and scientific history of Greek medical literature and medicine.

N.46), Cassius iatrosophista (II.22; N.46), Chariton (II.23), Constantinus Meliteniota (II.24; N.47), Damascenus (II.25), Eleutherus (II.35), Esdras propheta (II.37–38; N.50–51), Euphemius Siculus (II.38; N.51), Iacobus Psychrestus (II.50), Ioannes Chumnos (II.52), Ioannes Esdra (II.53), Ioannes episcopus Prisdyanesis (II.54; N.55), Ioannes Staphidaces (II.55; N.55), Leo (II.57; N.56), Manuel Comnenus (N.57), Maximus (Planudes?) (II.62; N.57), Neophytus Prodromenus (II.68; N.60), Nicolaus Myrepsus (II.69; N.60), Nicomedes iatrosophista (II.69), Paulus Nicaeensis (II.81; N.63), Perzoe (II.81), Philippus Xerus (N.63), Photius monachus (II.85),Taronitus (II.100; N.67), Theophilus (II.101–106; N.68), Theophylactus Simocata (II.106; N.68), and Ioannes Zacharias Actuarius (II.108–111; N.69).

43 Some *instrumenta studiorum* that might be considered as partial *New Diels* are already available. One of them is the catalogue of the manuscripts of the Latin translations of Hippocrates compiled by Pearl Kibre (above). Other two are the analytical lists of the manuscripts of the Arabic translations of Greek medical literature and original Arabic medical literature compiled by Sezgin 1970 (medicine, pharmacy, and zoology) and 1971 (alchemy, chemistry, botany, and agriculture), and Ullmann 1970 (medicine). One might also add the inventory of illustrated medical manuscripts compiled by MacKinney as early as 1965 (not only Greek and Latin, but also Syriac, Arabic and Turkish, and the roman languages, English, and German). Relevant also, the bibliographical lists compiled by Gerhard Fichtner (1932–2012) for Hippocrates and Galen (first published on demand, with several successive versions from 1985 on, and now available on line on the website of *Corpus Medicorum Graecorum*).

44 For a proposal in that sense, see Touwaide 2018. Whereas a publication upon completion of the research would be highly desirable, a gradual publication of available data in the form of a work in progress on the Internet might be useful, be it for a catalogue of manuscripts or a *New Diels*.

As such, the present work offers a set of new *instrumenta studiorum* for further developments in manuscript studies, the classical, medical and scientific traditions, and medical history.

Each of the five tomes of the present work has a specific content and purpose. The first tome exactly reproduces Diels' lists of Greek medical manuscripts[45], excluding the lists of the manuscripts containing the possible medieval translations of Greek medical texts into Syriac, Arabic, Hebrew, or Latin according to the treatises. It is not a photographic reproduction of Diels' original pages, however. Whereas lists of manuscripts in the original printing of Diels are presented in the form of blocks of continuous texts, they are rearranged here in the form of enumerations that clearly distinguish each item. The bibliography of Diels has been treated in a similar way for the purposes of clarity. The lists of manuscripts and the bibliography comprise most of the first tome, which is complemented by two indices: one of the authors and texts included in Diels, and the other of the manuscripts listed in Diels. For the purposes of easy and direct consultation, both of these indices open the first tome, which aims to not only make Diels available in a handy format, but to facilitate its use in research.

The remaining four tomes differ with regard to substance and purpose. All of them reproduce the contents of the manuscripts as described in Diels, including all annotations about title, *incipit*, *desinit* and lacunae, in addition to possible similarities with other manuscripts, sources, or copies. They proceed by manuscript (instead of by authors and works as in Diels' original publication). Identification of manuscripts exactly reproduces Diels' elements (city, library, and collection as appropriate, followed by shelfmark). The identification of many manuscripts required updating. This is the case for the several items known in Diels through earlier literature without exact identification. It is also the case of the codices destroyed during the two World Wars of the twentieth century, and of those that have changed location after the publication of Diels. Finally, it is also the case for those manuscripts which have received new shelfmarks. For all of these manuscripts, tomes two through five provide supplementary information with their exact identification, their state of preservation and location, or

---

45 Until a new reprint is published, Diels does not seem to be widely available (in spite of the 1970 reprint). WorldCat lists only 20 copies across the world. Nevertheless, digital copies are available on the Internet with different levels of quality, accuracy, and completeness via such sites as the *Corpus Medicorum Graecorum*, the Royal College of Physicians (RCP) in London, the Medic@ collection of the BIUSanté in Paris, the Digitale Bibliothek of the Münchener DigitalisierungsZentrum of the Bayerische Staatsbibliothek in Munich, and Google. These copies are linked on some other websites such as the Internet Archive, the UK Medical Heritage Library, the Medical Heritage Library, and European Libraries. As mentioned above, a database built on the basis of Diels is available on the website of the Institute for the Preservation of Medical Traditions.

their new shelfmark[46]. Another contribution of these tomes is their index of manuscripts, which includes possible new locations and shelfmarks, thus allowing one to search for manuscripts in two different, yet complementary ways: by their location and shelfmark as in Diels' time or in present time.

Besides these shared features, tomes two through five differ further by their content. Tomes two through four are each devoted to one author or a group of authors: tome two is devoted to Hippocrates, tome three to Galen, and tome four to the authors defined in Diels as *the remaining physicians* (*Die übrigen griechischen Ärzte ausser Galenos und Hippocrates*), that is, all the other authors of classical and late antiquity, with some Byzantine ones as well[47]. These three volumes aim to allow for a general study of the whole manuscript tradition of the textual bodies they are devoted to. Although they still have a limited documentary basis, they compensate for the lack of relevant instruments in currently available literature, and they provide the substance for first reconstructions of the whole tradition of the treatises by (or attributed to) Hippocrates, Galen, and the other Greek physicians considered by Diels.

Tome five goes further in laying down the basis of what will become a general catalogue of Greek medical manuscripts, as it lists the entire contents of all the manuscripts mentioned in Diels. It proceeds as do tomes two through four, by city and library in alphabetical order and, for each library, by collection and shelfmark, with their new locations and identifications as relevant. It also contains all the descriptive annotations about the texts included in Diels. Like tomes two through four, it contains an index of manuscripts that also lists possible new locations and identifications, allowing one to search for manuscripts on the basis of Diels or by their present location and identification.

By reproducing Diels' inventory of, and data on, Greek medical manuscripts, by rearranging them for new investigations, and by providing them with updated identification and new *instrumenta studiorum*, this work aims to not only make Diels newly available in a handy format with updated information and to expand the range of its applications, but to make further strides in the direction of a general catalogue of Greek medical manuscripts. This catalogue, in turn, will lead to the much needed *New Diels* that may be expected to transform the study and understanding of the Greek medical literature and medicine, with their tradition.

---

46 For these data, see Touwaide, 2016.

47 For these physicians, see note 42.

Bibliography

Ackermann 1791: Johannes Chr. Ackermann, "Caput XXIII De Hippocrate, Medicorum Principe, et Polybo eius Discipulo", in Ioannes Albertus Fabricius, *Bibliotheca Graeca sive Notitia Scriptorum Veterum Graecorum quorumcumque Monumenta Integra aut Fragmenta edita exstant tum plerorumque e MSS. ac deperditis ab auctore recognita.* Editio quarta variorum curis emendatior atque auctior curante Gottlieb Christophoro Harles. Accedunt B. I. A. Fabricii et Christoph. Augusti Heumanni Supplementa inedita, Volumen secundum. Hamburgi: apud Carolum Ernestum Bohn; Lipsiae: Ex Officina Breitkopfia, 1791, pp. 506–611.

Ackermann 1795: Johannes Chr. Ackermann, "Caput III De Dioscoride", in Ioannes Albertus Fabricius, *Bibliotheca Graeca sive Notitia Scriptorum Veterum Graecorum quorumcumque Monumenta Integra aut Fragmenta edita exstant tum plerorumque e MSS. ac deperditis ab auctore recognita.* Editio tertia variorum curis emendatior atque auctior curante Gottlieb Christophoro Harles. Accedunt Christophori Augusti Heumanni Supplementa inedita, Volumen quartum. Hamburgi: apud Carolum Ernestum Bohn; Lipsiae: Ex Officina Breitkopfia et Haertelia, 1795, pp. 673–702.

Ackermann 1796: Johannes Chr. Ackermann, " Caput XIX (olim XVII) Claudius Galenus", in Ioannes Albertus Fabricius, *Bibliotheca Graeca sive Notitia Scriptorum Veterum Graecorum quorumcumque Monumenta Integra aut Fragmenta edita exstant tum plerorumque e MSS. ac deperditis ab auctore recognita.* Editio tertia variorum curis emendatior atque auctior curante Gottlieb Christophoro Harles. Accedunt Christophori Augusti Heumanni Supplementa inedita, Volumen quintum. Hamburgi: apud Carolum Ernestum Bohn; Lipsiae: Ex Officina Breitkopfia et Haertelia, 1796, pp. 377–500.

Ackermann 1821: Johannes Chr. Ackermann, "Historia literaria Claudii Galeni ... ex Jo. Alb. Fabricii Biblioth. Graec. ex ed. Gli. Cph. Harles, vol. V. P. 377–500", in Carolus Gottlob Kühn (ed.), *Claudii Galeni Opera omnia*, Tomus 1 (Medicorum Graecorum Opera quae exstant 1). Leipzig: Carl Cnobloch, 1821, pp. XVII–CCLXV.

Ackermann 1825: Johannes Chr. Ackermann, "Historia literaria Hippocratis ... ex Jo. Alb. Fabricii Biblioth. Graec. ex edit. Gli. Cph. Harles, vol. II. P. 506–511. Desunta et hinc inde aucta et emendata", in Carolus Gottlob Kühn (ed.), *Magni Hippocratis Opera omnia*, Tomus 1 (Medicorum Graecorum Opera quae exstant 21). Leipzig: Carl Cnobloch, 1825, pp. I–CCVI).

Alexanderson 1963: Bengt Alexanderson, *Die Hippokratische Schrift Prognostikon. Überlieferung and Text* (Studia Graeca et Latina Gothoburgensia 17). Göteborg: Acta Universitatis Gothoburgensis, 1963.

Alexanderson 1967: Bengt Alexanderson, *Galenos, Περὶ κρίσεων. Uberlieferung und Text* (Studia Graeca et Latina Gothoburgensia 23). Göteborg: Acta Universitatis Gothoburgensis, 1967.

Bennett 2016: David Bennett, *Medicine and Pharmacy in Byzantine Hospitals. A study of the extant formularies* (Medicine in the Medieval Mediterranean 7). London and New York, NY: Routledge, 2016.

Bersgträsser 1914: Gotthelf Bergsträsser (ed.), *Pseudogaleni in Hippocratis de septimanis* (Corpus Medicorum Graecorum XI 2,1). Lipsiae et Berolini: B.G. Teubner, 1914.

Bernabò 2010: Massimo Bernabò (ed.), *La collezione di testi chirurgici di Niceta. Firenze, Biblioteca Medicea Laurenziana, plut. 74.7. Tradizione medica classica a Bisanzio* (Folia Picta. Manoscritti miniati medievali 2). Roma: Storia e Letteratura, 2010.

Boudon 2000: Véronique Boudon, *Galien*, Tome II: *Exhortation à l'étude de la médecine. Art médical.* Texte établi et traduit (Collection des Universités de France). Paris: Belles Lettres, 2000.

Bouras-Vallianatos 2015: Petros Bouras-Vallianatos, "Greek Manuscripts at the Wellcome Library in London: A Descriptive Catalogue", *Medical History* 59 (2015), pp. 275–326.

Bouras-Vallianatos 2020: Petros Bouras-Vallianatos, "Addenda et Corrigenda to the 'Greek Manuscripts at the Wellcome Library in London: A Descriptive Catalogue', *Medical History* 59 (2015): 275–326", in Petros Bouras-Vallianatos (ed.), *Exploring Greek Manuscripts in the Library at Wellcome Collection in London*. London: Routledge, 2020, pp. 181–182.

Calder et al. 1999: William M. Calder III, and Jaap Mansfeld (eds.), with the participation of Alex Leukart, François Paschould, and Olivier Reverdin, *Hermann Diels (1848–1922) et la science de l'Antiquité. Huit exposés suivis de discussion ... Vandoeuvres-Genève, 17–21 août 1998* (Entretiens sur l'Antiquité classique 45). Genève: Fondation Hardt, 1999.

Cavallo 1988: Guglielmo Cavallo, *Le biblioteche nel mondo antico e medievale* (Biblioteca universale Laterza 250). Bari and Roma: Laterza, 1988.

Cavallo 1993: Guglielmo Cavallo, "Libri di medicina: gli usi di un sapere", in Evelyne Patlagean (ed.), *Maladie et société à Byzance* (Collectanea 3). Spoleto: Centro italiano di studi sull'alto medioevo, 1993, pp. 43–56.

Cavallo and Chartier 1995: Guglielmo Cavallo and Roger Chartier (eds), *Storia della lettura nel mondo occidentale* (Storia e Società). Bari and Roma: Laterza, 1995.

Chatzopoulou 2014: Βενετία Χατζοπούλου, "Δύο ἄγνωστα ἰατρικά χειρόγραφα μὲ ἔργα τοῦ Νικολάου Βελισδονίτη", in Παναγιώτης Βλάχος, *Όσιος Ευγένιος ο Αιτωλός και αι Σχολαί των Αγράφων κατά την Τουρκοκρατία. Καρπενήσιον, 7–9 Ὀκτωβρίου 2011. Πρακτικά*. Αθήνα: Σύνδεσμος "Ευγένιος ο Αιτωλός", 2014, vol. 2, pp. 573–581.

Clark 2011: Patricia A. Clark, *A Cretan Healer's Handbook in the Byzantine Tradition: Text, Translation and Commentary* (Medicine in the Medieval Mediterranean 3). Aldershot, and Burlington, VT: Ashgate, 2011.

Costomiris 1889: Georges A. Costomiris, "Etudes sur les écrits inédits des anciens médecins grecs et ceux dont le texte original est perdu, mais qui existent en latin ou en arabe. Première série: Hippocrate, Cratevas, Aelius Promotus, Galien", *Revue des études grecques* 1 (1889), pp. 343–383.

Costomiris 1890: Georges A. Costomiris, "Etudes sur les écrits inédits des anciens médecins grecs et ceux dont le texte original est perdu, mais qui existent en latin ou en arabe. Deuxième série: L'Anonyme de Daremberg, Métrodora, Aétius", *Revue des études grecques* 3 (1890), pp. 145–179.

Costomiris 1891: Georges A. Costomiris, "Etudes sur les écrits inédits des anciens médecins grecs et ceux dont le texte original est perdu, mais qui existent en latin ou en arabe. Troisième série: Alexandre (Sophiste et Roi), Timothée, Léon le Sophiste, Théophane Nonnos, les Ephodes", *Revue des études grecques* 4 (1891), pp. 97–110.

Costomiris 1892: Georges A. Costomiris, "Études sur les écrits inédits des anciens médecins grecs. Quatrième série: Hippiatriques et auteurs du XIe siècle: Psellus, Siméon Seth, Damnastès", *Revue des études grecques*, 5 (1892), pp. 61–72.

Costomiris 1897: Georges A. Costomiris, "Etudes sur les écrits inédits des anciens médecins grecs et ceux dont le texte original est perdu, mais qui existent en latin ou en arabe. Cinquième série: XIIIe–XIVe siècles, Jean Tzetzès, Nicolas Myrepsus, Jean Actuarius", *Revue des études grecques* 10 (1897), pp. 405–445.

Dain 1930: Alphonse Dain, *Les manuscrits d'Onesandros* (Collection d'études anciennes). Paris: Belles Lettres, 1930.

Dain 1933: Alphonse Dain, *La tradition du texte d'Héron de Byzance* (Collection d'études anciennes). Paris: Belles Lettres, 1933.

Dain 1946: Alphonse Dain, *Histoire du texte d'Élien le Tacticien des origines à la fin du moyen âge* (Collection d'études anciennes). Paris: Belles Lettres, 1946.

Dain 1949: Alphonse Dain, *Les manuscrits*. Paris: Belles Lettes, 1949.

Daremberg 1845: Charles Daremberg, "Rapport adressé à M. le Ministre de l'Instruction Publique par .. chargé d'une mission médico-littéraire en Allemagne" *Journal général de l'Instruction publique* 14, no. 33 (23 avril 1845), pp. 193–196, and no. 34 (26 avril 1845), pp. 198–202 (also printed as a booklet under the same title, in Paris, P. Dupont, 15 avril 1845, 32 p.).

Daremberg 1848: Charles Daremberg, "Résumé d'un voyage médico-littéraire en Angleterre. Lu à l'Académie des inscriptions et belle-lettres, dans la séance du 6 octobre", *Gazette médicale de Paris*, 4 novembre 1848, pp. 3–18.

Daremberg 1851: Charles Daremberg, "Notices et extraites des manuscrits médicaux d'Angleterre", *Archives des Missions scientifiques et littéraires*, 1851,VII, VIII, and IX.

Daremberg 1852: Charles Daremberg, "Notices et extraites des manuscrits médicaux d'Angleterre", *Archives des Missions scientifiques et littéraires* 1852, I.

Daremberg 1853: Charles Daremberg, *Notices et extraits des manuscrits médicaux grecs, latins et français, des principales bibliothèques de l'Europe, I: Manuscrits grecs d'Angleterre suivis d'un fragment de Gilles de Corbeil et de scolies inédites sur Hippocrate*. Paris: Imprimerie impériale, 1853.

De Boer 1937: Wilko De Boer (ed.), *Galeni De propriorum animi cuiuslibet dignotione et curatione. De animi cuiuslibet peccatorum dignotione et curatione. De atra bile* (Corpus Medicorum Graecorum V 4, 1. 1). Lipsiae et Berolini: B. G. Teubner, 1937.

Dickson 1998: Keith Dickson (ed.), *Stephanus the Philosopher and Physician, Commentary on Galen's Therapeutics to Glaucon* (Studies in Ancient Medicine 19). Leiden, Boston, MA, Köln: Brill, 1998.

Diels 1905: Hermann Diels (ed.), *Die Handschriften der antiken Ärzte. I. Teil. Hippokrates und Galenos. Im Auftrage der akademischen Kommission herausgegeben* (Abhandlungen der Königlich Preussischen Akademie der Wissenschaften vom Jahre 1905, Philosophisch-historische Klasse, Abhandlung III). Berlin: Königliche Akademie der Wissenschaften, 1905.

Diels 1906a: Hermann Diels, *Die Handschriften der antiken Ärzte. II. Teil. Die übrigen griechischen Ärzte ausser Hippokrates und Galenos. Im Auftrage der akademischen Kommission herausgegeben von -* (Abhandlungen der Königlich Preussischen Akademie der Wissenschaften vom Jahre 1906, Philosophisch-historische Klasse, Abhandlung I). Berlin: Königliche Akademie der Wissenschaften, 1906.

Diels 1906b: Hermann Diels, *Die Handschriften der antiken Ärzte. Griechische Abteilung. Im Auftrage der akademischen Kommission herausgegeben von - aus den Abhandlungen der Königlich Preussischen Akademie der Wissenschaften der Jahre 1905 und 1906*. Berlin: Königliche Akademie der Wissenschaften, 1906.

Diels 1908: Hermann Diels, *Bericht über den Stand des interakademischen Corpus Medicorum Antiquorum und Erster Nachtrag zu den in den Abhandlungen 1905 und 1906 veröffentlichten Katalogen: Die Handschriften der antiken Ärzte. I. und II. Teil. Zusammengestellt im Namen der Kommission der Königlich Preussischen Akademie der Wissenschaften von -* (Abhandlungen der Königlich Preussischen Akademie der Wissenschaften vom Jahre 1907, Philosophisch-historische Klasse, Abhandlung II). Berlin: Königliche Akademie der Wissenschaften, 1908.

Diels 1912: Hermann Diels, *Die handschriftliche Überlieferung des galenischen Commentars zum Prorrheticum des Hippocrates* (Abhandlungen der Königlich Preussischen Akademie der Wissenschaften vom Jahre 1912, Philosophisch-historische Klasse, Abhandlung I). Berlin: Königliche Akademie der Wissenschaften, 1912.

Diels et al. 1915: Hermann Diels (ed.), *Galeni, In Hippocratis Prorrheticum I commentaria III*; Johannes Mewaldt (ed.), *Galeni, De comate secundum Hippocratem*; Josef Heeg (ed.), *Galeni, In Hippocratis Prognosticum commentaria III* (Corpus Medicorum Graecorum V 9, 2). Lipsiae et Berolini: B. G. Teubneri, 1915.

Dietz 1832: Friedrich Reinhold Dietz, *Galeni de dissectione musculorum et de consuetudine libri. Ad fidem codicum manuscriptorum alterum secundum, primum alterum graece edidit.* Lipsiae: Leopold Voss, 1832.

Dietz 1834: Friedrich Reinhold Dietz, *Apollonii Citiensis, Stephani, Palladii, Theophili, Meletii, Damasci, Ioannis aliorum Scholia in Hippocratem et Galenum e codicibus mss. Vindobonens. Monacens. Florentin. Mediolanens. Escorialens. etc. primum graece edidit*, 2 volumes. Regimontii Prussorum: apud fratres Borntraeger, 1834.

Dietz 1836: Friedrich Reinhold Dietz, *Severi Iatrosophistae De clysteribus liber. Ad Fidem Codicis Manuscripti unici Florentini primum Graece edidit.* Regimontii Prussorum: apud Fratres Borntraeger, 1836.

Dumouchel 1995: Paul Dumouchel, *Emotions. Essai sur le corps et le social* (Collection Les Empêcheurs de penser en rond). Le Plessis-Robinson: Synthélabo, 1995.

Durling 1967: Richard J. Durling, "Corrigenda and addenda to Diels' Galenica. I. Codices Vaticani". *Traditio* 23 (1967), pp. 461–476.

Durling 1981: Richard J. Durling, "Corrigenda and addenda to Diels' Galenica. II. Codices Miscellanei". *Traditio* 37 (1981), pp. 373–381.

Durling 1985–1993: Richard J. Durling, "A Guide to the Medical Manuscripts Mentioned in Kristeller's *Iter Italicum*", *Traditio* 41 (1985), pp. 341–365; 44 (1988), pp. 485–536; 46 (1991), pp. 347–379; 48 (1993), pp. 253–316.

Eleuteri 1981: Paolo Eleuteri, *Storia della tradizione manoscritta di Museo* (Biblioteca di Studi Antichi 30). Pisa: Giardini, 1981.

Fabricius 1705–1728: Jo. Alberti Fabricii, *Bibliotheca Graeca* ... Hamburgi: Sumptu Christiani Lievezeit, Typis Spiringlanis, 1705–1728, 14 volumes (after the general title as above, each volume has a specific subtitle that details its contents).

Fabricius ed. Harles 1790–1838: Gottlieb Christophorus Harles, *Ioannis Alberti Fabricii ... Bibliotheca Graeca sive notitia scriptorum veterum graecorum quorumcunque monumenta integra aut fragmenta edita exstant tum plerorumque e MSS. ac deperditis ab auctore tertium recognita et plurimis locis aucta editio quarta variorum curis emendatior atque auctior ... Accedunt B. I. A. Fabricii et Christoph. Augusti Heumanni supplementa inedita.* Hamburgi: apud Carolum Ernestum Bohn; Lipsiae: ex Officina Breitkoppia, 1790–1838, 13 volumes.

Fichtner 1985a: Gerhard Fichtner, *Corpus Galenicum. Verzeichnis der galenischen und pseudogalenischen Schriften.* Tübingen: the author, 1985.

Fichtner 1985b: Gerhard Fichtner, *Corpus Hippocraticum. Verzeichnis der hippokratischen und pseudohippokratischen Schriften.* Tübingen: the author, 1985.

Fischer 1991: Jean-Louis Fischer, *Monstres. Histoire du corps et de ses défauts.* Paris: Syros Alternatives, 1991.

Formentin 1978: Mariarosa Formentin, *I codici greci di medicina nelle tre Venezie* (Università di Padova, Studi bizantini e neogreci 10). Padova: Liviana editrice, 1978.

Formentin 1997: Maria Rosa Formentin, "Codici greci di medicina nella Biblioteca Nazionale Vittorio Emanuele III di Napoli: le vie di acquisizione", in Sergio Sconocchia and Lucio Toneatto (eds.), in collaboration with Daria Crismani, Michele Faraguna, and Italo Pin, *Lingue tecniche del greco e del latino II. Atti del II Seminario internazionale sulla letteratura scientifica e tecnica greca e latina (Trieste, 4–5 ottobre 1993).* Bologna: Pàtron, 1997, pp. 208–216.

Fortuna and Raia 2006: Stefania Fortuna and Annamaria Raia, "Corrigenda and Addenda to Diels *Galenica* by Richard J. Durling: III. Manuscripts and Editions", *Traditio* 61 (2006), pp. 1–30.

Garzya 1992: Antonio Garzya (ed.), *Tradizione e ecdotica dei testi medici tardo-antichi e bizantini. Atti del Convegno internazionale, Anacapri, 29–31 ottobre 1990* (Collectanea 5). Napoli: D'Auria, 1992.

Garzya and Masullo 2004: Antonio Garzya and Rita Masullo (eds), *I problemi di Cassio Iatrosofista. Testo critico, introduzione, apparato critico, traduzione e note.* Napoli: Accademia Pontaniana, 2004.

Green 1996: Monica H. Green, "A Handlist of the Latin and Vernacular Manuscripts of the So-Called Trotula Texts. Part I: The Latin Manuscripts", *Scriptorium* 50 (1996), pp. 137–175.

Green 1997: Monica H. Green, "A Handlist of the Latin and Vernacular Manuscripts of the So-Called Trotula Texts. Part II: The Vernacular Texts and Latin Re-Writings", *Scriptorium* 51 (1997), pp. 80–104.

Haller 1771–1772: Albrecht von Haller, *Bibliotheca botanica qua scripta ad rem herbariam facientia a rerum initiis recensentur*, 2 volumes. Tiguri: Orell, Gessner, Fuessli, et Socc., 1771–1772.

Haller 1774–1775: Albrecht von Haller, *Bibliotheca chirurgica qua scripta ad artem chirurgicam facientia a rerum initiis recensentur*, 2 volumes. Bernae: Em. Haller; Basileae: Joh. Schweighauser, 1774–1775.

Haller 1774–1777: Albrecht von Haller, *Bibliotheca anatomica qua scripta ad anatomen et physiologiam facientia a rerum initiis recensentur*, 2 volumes. Tiguri: Orell, Gessner, Fuessli, et Socc., 1774–1777.

Haller 1776–1788: Albrecht von Haller, *Bibliotheca medicinae practicae qua scripta ad partem medicinae practicam facientia a rerum initiis ad A. MDCCLXXV recensentur*, 4 volumes. Basileae: Joh. Schweighauser, and Bernae: Em. Haller, 1776–1788.

Heiberg 1921–1924: Johannes L. Heiberg (ed.), *Paulus Aegineta*, 2 volumes (Corpus Medicorum Graecorum IX 1–2). Lipsiae et Berolini: B. G. Teubner, 1921–1924.

Heiberg et al. 1927: Johannes L. Heiberg, Johannes Mewaldt, Ernst Nachmanson, Hermann Schoene (eds), *Hippocratis opera: Indices librorum, Iusiurandum, Lex, De arte, De medico, De decente habitu, Praeceptiones, De prisca medicina, De aere locis aquis, De alimento, De liquidorum usu, De flatibus* (Corpus Medicorum Graecorum I 1). Lipsiae et Berolini: B. G. Teubner, 1927.

Helmreich 1913: Georg Helmreich, *Handschriftliche Studien zu Symeon Seth* (Programm des K. humanistischen Gymnasiums in Ansbach für das Schuljahr 1912/13). Ansbach: C. Brügel & Sohn, 1913.

Henry 1938: Paul Henry, *Études Plotiniennes I. Les Etats du texte de Plotin* (Museum Lessianum, Section Philosophique, no 20). Paris: Desclée de Brouwer et Cie; Bruxelles: L'Edition Universelle, 1938.

Henry 1941: Paul Henry, *Études Plotiniennes II. Les Manuscrits des Ennéades* (Museum Lessianum, Section Philosophique 21). Bruxelles: L'Edition Universelle; Paris: Desclée de Brouwer et Cie, and A. et J. Picard, 1941.

Herida 1998: Magid Herida, *La peau dans les écrits hippocratiques* (Thèse de médecine). Paris: Université Paris 6, 1998.

Hunger and Kresten 1969: Herbert Hunger, and Otto Kresten, *Katalog der griechischen Handschriften der Österreichischen Nationalbibliothek*, Teil 2: *Codices juridici, codices medici* (Museion, Veröffentlichungen der Österreichischen Nationalbibliothek, Neue Folge, Vierte Reihe: Veröffentlichungen der Handschriftensammlung, Erster Band: Katalog der griechischen Handschriften der Österreichischen Nationalbibliothek, Teil 2). Wien: Georg Prachner, 1969.

Ieraci Bio 1989: Anna Maria Ieraci Bio, "La trasmissione della letteratura medica greca nell'Italia meridionale fra X e XV secolo", in Antonio Garzya (ed.), *Contributi alla cultura greca nell'Italia meridionale* (Hellenica et Byzantina Neapolitana 13). Napoli: Bibliopolis, 1989, pp. 133–257.

Ihm 2002: Sibylle Ihm, *Clavis Commentariorum der antiken medizinischen Texte* (Clavis Commentariorum Antiquitatis et Medii Aevi 1). Leiden, Boston and Köln: Brill, 2002.

Ilberg 1911: Johannes Ilberg, *Die Überlieferung der Gynäkologie des Soranos von Ephesos* (Abhandlungen der philologisch-historischen Klasse der Königl. Sächsischen Gesellschaft der Wissenschaften Bd. 28, Abhandlung 2). Leipzig: B. G. Teubner, 1911.

Ilberg 1927: Ioannes Ilberg (ed.), *Soranus* (Corpus Medicorum Graecorum IV). Lipsiae et Berolini: B. G. Teubner, 1927.

Irigoin 1952: Jean Irigoin, *Histoire du Texte de Pindare* (Etudes et Commentaires 13). Paris: Klincksieck, 1952.

Irigoin 1970: Jean Irigoin, "Les manuscrits grecs. I. Quelques catalogues récents", *Revue des études grecques* 83 (1970), pp. 500–529.

Joly 1978: Robert Joly, *Hippocrate. Oeuvres complètes*, Tome XIII: *Les lieux dans l'homme. Du système des glandes. Des fistules. Des hémorrhoïdes. De la vision. Des chairs. De la dentition*. Texte établi et traduit (Collection des Universités de France). Paris: Belles Lettres, 1978.

Karas 1994: Γιάννης Καράς, *Οι επιστήμες στην Τουρκοκρατία. Χειρόγραφα και έντυπα*, Τόμος Γ': Οι επιστήμες της ζώης. Παράρτημα. Έργα γενικόν γνωσέων (Κέντρο Νεοελληνικών Ερευνών, Έθνικό Ίδρυμα Ερευνών 48). Αθήνα: Βιβλιοπωλείον της «Εστίας», 1994.

Kibre 1975–1982: Pearl Kibre, "Hippocrates Latinus. Repertorium of Hippocratic Writings in the Latin Middle Ages", *Traditio* 31 (1975), pp. 99–126; 32 (1976), pp. 257–292; 33 (1977), pp. 253–295; 34 (1978), pp. 193–226; 35 (1979), pp. 273–302; 36 (1980), pp. 347–392; 37 (1981), pp. 267–289; 38 (1982), pp. 165–192.

Kibre 1985: Pearl Kibre, *Hippocrates Latinus. Repertorium of Hippocratic Writings in the Latin Middle Ages*. Revised Edition. New York: Fordham University Press, 1985.

Koch et al. 1923: Konrad Koch (ed.), *Galeni, De sanitate tuenda libri VI*; Georg Helmreich (ed.), *Galeni, De alimentorum facultatibus libri III*; *Galeni, De bonis malisque sucis lber*; Karl Kalbfleisch (ed.), *Galeni, De victu attenuante*; Otto Hartlich (ed.), *Galeni, De ptisana* (Corpus Medicorum Graecorum V 4, 2). Lipsiae et Berolini: B. G. Teubner, 1923.

Kollesch 1973: Jutta Kollesch, "Hermann Diels in seiner Bedeutung für die Geschichte der antiken Medizin", *Philologus* 117 (1973), pp. 278–283.

Kollesch 1989: "Die Erschliessung der antiken medizinischen Texte und ihre Probleme – das *Corpus Medicorum Graecorum et Latinorum*", *Gesnerus* 46 (1989), pp. 195–210.

Kollesch 1999: "Die Organisation und Herausgabe des *Corpus Medicorum Graecorum*: ergänzenden Details aus der Korrespondenz zwischen Hermann Diels und Johannes Mewaldt", in William M. Calder III, and Jaap Mansfeld (eds.), with the participation of Alex Leukart, François Paschould, and Olivier Reverdin, *Hermann Diels (1848–1922) et la science de l'Antiquité. Huit exposés suivis de discussion ... Vandoeuvres-Genève, 17–21 août 1998* (Entretiens sur l'Antiquité classique 45). Genève: Fondation Hardt, 1999, pp. 207–223.

Kudlien 1960: Fridolf Kudlien, *Die handschriftliche Überlieferung des Galenkommentars zu Hippokrates de articulis* (Deutsche Akademie der Wissenschaften zu Berlin, Schriften der Sektion für Altertumswissenschaft 27). Berlin: Akademie Verlag, 1960.

Kudlien 1970: Fridolf Kudlien (ed.), *Hermann Alexander Diels, Die Handschriften der antiken Ärzte. I Hippokrates und Galenos II Die übrigen griechische Ärzte III Nachtrag*. Mit einem Vorwort. Leipzig: Zentralantiquariat der deutschen demokratischen Republik, 1970.

Kühn 1821: Karl Gottlieb Kühn (ed.), *Claudii Galeni Opera omnia*, Tomus I (Medicorum graecorum opera quae exstant 1). Lipsiae: Cnobloch, 1821.

Kühn 1825: Karl Gottlieb Kühn (ed.), *Magni Hippocratis Opera omnia*, Tomus I (Medicorum graecorum opera quae exstant 21). Lipsiae: Cnobloch, 1825.

Lamagna 2017: Mario Lamagna, *Giovanni Attuario, L'eccellente trattato sulle urine di Avicenna*. Introduzione, testo critico, traduzione e note al testo (Serie Textos Médicos – Ediciones Críticas.

Ediciones críticas de la Escuela de traductores de Toledo 21). Cuenca: Ediciones de la Universidad de Castilla-La Mancha, 2017.

MacKinney 1965: Loren MacKinney, *Medical Illustrations in Medieval Manuscripts* (Publications of the Wellcome Historical Medical Library, New Series, V). London: Wellcome Historical Medical Library, 1965.

Marx 1915: Fridericus Marx (ed.), *A. Cornelii Celsi quae supersunt* (Corpus Medicorum Latinorum I). Lipsiae et Berolini: In aedibus B. G. Teubneri, 1915.

Masullo 2006: Rita Masullo, "Sul ΠΕΡΙ ΣΦΥΓΜΩΝ attribuito a Mercurio Monaco", in Véronique Boudon-Millot, Antonio Garzya, Jacques Jouanna, and Amneris Roselli (eds.), *Ecdotica e ricezione dei testi medici greci. Atti del V Convegno Internazionale Napoli, 1–2 ottobre 2004* (Collectanea 24). Napoli: M. D'Auria, 2006, pp. 335–346.

Mewaldt et al. 1914: Johannes Mewaldt (ed.), *Galeni, In Hippocratis De natura hominis commentaria III*; Georg Helmreich (ed.), *Galeni, In Hippocratis De victu acutorum commentaria IV*; Johann Westenberger (ed.), *Galeni, De diaeta Hippocratis in morbis acutis* (Corpus Medicorum Graecorum V 9, 1). Lipsiae et Berolini: B. G. Teubner, 1914.

Mercati 1916: Giovanni Mercati, "Minuzie. – 6–8. Pretesi scritti di Paolo l'Egineta e di Galeno. – 9–11. Pretesi scritti di medicina greca", *Bessarione* 32 (1916), pp. 208–211 (reprinted in Giovanni Mercati, *Opere minori raccolte in occasione del settantesimo natalizio sotto gli auspicii di S. S. Pio XI*, vol. 3 [1907–1916] (Studi e Testi 780. Città del Vaticano: Biblioteca Apostolica Vaticana, 1937, pp. 521–524).

Mercati 1917a: Giovanni Mercati, "Minuzie. – 13–17. Altre correzioni ed aggiunte all'op. Die Handschriften der antiken Aerzte. – 18. Per Aezio", *Bessarione* 38 (1917), pp. 50–55 (reprinted in Giovanni Mercati, *Opere minori raccolte in occasione del settantesimo natalizio sotto gli auspicii di S. S. Pio XI*, vol. 4 [1917–1936] (Studi e Testi 79). Città del Vaticano: Biblioteca Apostolica Vaticana, 1937, pp. 16–21).

Mercati 1917b: Giovanni Mercati, "I. Filippo Xeros Reggino, Giovanni Alessandrino iatrosofista e altri nel codice Vaticano degli Ephodia, and II. Un nuovo capitolo di Sorano e tre nuove ricette superstiziose in Aezio", in Giovanni Mercati, *Notizie varie di antica letteratura medica e di bibliografia* (Studi e Testi 31). Roma: Tipografia Poliglotta Vaticana, 1917, pp. 9–41, and 42–46.

Mondrain 2003: Brigitte Mondrain, "Comment était lu Galien à Byzance dans la première moitié du XVe siècle? Contribution à quelques aspects de l'histoire des textes", in Antonio Garzya and Jacques Jouanna (eds), *Trasmissione e ecdotica dei testi medici greci. Atti del IV Convegno internazionale, Parigi 17–19 maggio 2001* (Collectanea 21). Napoli: D'Auria, 2003, pp. 361–384.

Morani 1981: Moreno Morani, *La tradizione manoscritta del "De natura hominis" di Nemesio* (Scienze filologiche e letteratura 18). Milano: Vita e pensiero, 1981.

Nutton 2004: Vivian Nutton, "Ancient Medicine: From Berlin to Baltimore", in Frank Huisman, and John Harley Warner (eds), *Locating Medical History. The Stories and Their Meanings*. Baltimore, MD, and London: Johns Hopkins University Press, 2004, pp. 115–138.

Olivier 1995: Jean-Marie Olivier, *Répertoire des bibliothèques et des catalogues de manuscrits grecs de Marcel Richard. Troisième édition entièrement refondue* (Corpus Christianorum). Turnhout: Brepols, 1995.

Olivier 2018: Jean-Marie Olivier, *Supplément au répertoire des bibliothèques et des catalogues de manuscrits grecs*, 2 volumes (Corpus Christianorum). Turnhout: Brepols, 2018.

Olivieri 1935: Alessandro Olivieri (ed.), *Aetii Amideni Libri medicinales I–IV* (Corpus Medicorum Graecorum VIII 1). Lipsiae et Berolini: B. G. Teubner, 1935.

***Paléographie* 1977:** *La paléographie grecque et byzantine: actes du colloque international sur la paléographie grecque et byzantine organisé dans le cadre des colloques internationaux du Centre*

National de la recherche scientifique, Paris du 21 au 25 octobre 1974 (Issue 559 of Colloques internationaux du Centre National de la Recherche Scientifique 559). Paris: Editions du CNRS, 1977.

Perilli 1999: Lorenzo Perilli, "La tradizione manoscritta del Glossario ippocratico di Galeno (e l'ordinamento alfabetico delle glosse)", in Antonio Garzya, and Jacques Jouanna (eds.), *I testi medici greci. Tradizione e ecdotica. Atti del III Convegno Internazionale, Napoli 15–18 ottobre 1997*. Napoli: M. D'Auria, 1999, pp. 429–456.

Perilli 2011: Lorenzo Perilli, "Nuovi manoscritti del Glossario Ippocratico di Galeno e considerazioni stemmatiche. *Codex olim Mosquensis, codex Bodleianus Holkhamensis 92*", in Lorenzo Perilli, Christian Brockmann, Klaus-Dietrich Fischer, and Amneris Roselli (eds), *Officina Hippocratica. Beiträge zu Ehren von Anargyros Anastassiou und Dieter Irmer* (Beiträge zur Altertumskunde 289). Berlin and Boston, MA: De Gruyter, 2011, pp. 177–201.

Perrin 1988: Christophe Perrin, *La peau ou la représentation du corps malade: médecines antiques, médecine anatomo-clinique* (Thèse médecine) Nice: Université de Nice, 1988.

Petit 2006: Caroline Petit, "Les manuscrits de Modène et la tradition de l'*Introductio sive medicus* du Pseudo-Galien", in Véronique Boudon-Millot, Antonio Garzya, Jacques Jouanna, and Amneris Roselli (eds), *Ecdotica e ricezione dei testi medici greci. Atti del V Convegno Internazionale, Napoli, 1–2 ottobre 2004* (Collectanea 24). Napoli: M. D'Auria, 2006, pp. 167–185.

Pietrobelli 2010: Antoine Pietrobelli, "Variation autour du Thessalonicensis Vlatadon 14: un manuscrit copié au Xénon du Kral, peu avant la chute de Constantinople", *Revue des études byzantines* 68 (2010), pp. 95–126.

Pritchet 1975: Christopher Dixon Pritchet (ed.), *Iohannis Alexandrini Commentaria in sextum librum Hippocratis Epidemiarum recognovit et adnotatione critica instruxit*. Leiden: Brill, 1975.

Pritchet 1982: Christopher Dixon Pritchet (ed.), *Iohannis Alexandrini Commentaria in librum De sectis Galeni*. Recognovit et adnotatione critica instruxit. Leiden: E. J. Brill, 1982.

Raeder 1926: Ioannes Raeder (ed.), *Oribasii, Synopsis ad Eustathium; Libri ad Eunapium* (Corpus Medicorum Graecorum VI 3). Lipsiae et Berolini: B. G. Teubner, 1926.

Raeder 1928–1933: Ioannes Raeder (ed.), *Oribasii, Collectionum medicarum reliquiae*, 4 volumes (Corpus Medicorum Graecorum VI 1, 1–2; VI 2, 1–2). Lipsiae et Berolini: B. G. Teubner, 1928–1933.

Regling 1920: Kurt Regling, "Bruno Rappaport. Geb. den 4. November 1875, gest. den 20. Juli 1915", *Biographisches Jahrbuch für die Altertumswissenschaft* 40 (1920), pp. 76–83.

Rey 1993: Roselyne Rey, *Histoire de la douleur* (Histoire des sciences). Paris: La Découverte, 1993.

Richard 1948: Marcel Richard, *Répertoire des bibliothèques et des catalogues de nanuscrits grecs* (Publications de l'Institut de recherche et d'histoire des textes 1). Paris: Centre de documentation du Centre National de la Recherche Scientifique, 1948.

Richard 1958: Marcel Richard, *Répertoire des bibliothèques et des catalogues de manuscrits grecs*. Deuxième édition (Centre national de la recherche scientifique, Publications de l'Institut de recherche et d'histoire des textes 1). Paris: Centre national de la recherche scientifique, 1958.

Richard 1964: Marcel Richard, *Répertoire des bibliothèques et des catalogues de manuscrits grecs. Supplément I (1958–1963)* (Documents, études et répertoires publiés par l'Institut de recherche et d'histoire des textes 9). Paris: Éditions du Centre National de la Recherche Scientifique, 1964.

Rivier 1962: André Rivier, *Recherches sur la tradition manuscrite du traité hippocratique "De morbo sacro"* (Travaux publiés sous les auspices de la Société suisse des sciences morales 3). Berne: Francke, 1962.

Roselli 2009: Amneris Roselli, "Due manoscritti medici greci nelle biblioteche di Sofia", *Galenos* 3 (2009), pp. 177–180.

Sarton 1927–1948: George Sarton, *Introduction to the History of Science*, 3 volumes in five tomes. Baltimore: Williams & Wilkins, 1927–1948.

Sezgin 1970: Fuat Sezgin, *Geschichte des arabischen Schrifttums*, Band 3: *Medizin, Pharmazie, Zoologie, Tierheilkunde bis ca. 430 H.* Leiden: E.J.Brill, 1970.

Sezgin 1971: Fuat Sezgin, *Geschichte des arabischen Schrifttums*, Band 4: *Alchimie, Chemie, Botanik, Agrikultur bis ca. 430 H.* Leiden: E.J.Brill, 1971.

Sinkewicz 1990: Robert E. Sinkewicz, *Manuscript Listings for the Authors of Classical and Late Antiquity* (Greek Index Project Series 3). Toronto: Pontifical Institute of Mediaeval Studies, 1990.

Sinkewicz 1992: Robert E. Sinkewicz, *Manuscript Listings for the Authors of the Patristic and Byzantine Periods* (Greek Index Project Series 4). Toronto: Pontifical Institute of Mediaeval Studies, 1992.

Sinkewicz and Hayes 1989: Robert E. Sinkewicz and Walter H. Hayes, *Manuscript Listings for the Authored Works of the Palaeologan Period* (Greek Index Project Series 2). Toronto: Pontifical Institute of Mediaeval Studies, 1989.

Sonderkamp 1987: Joseph A. M. Sonderkamp, *Untersuchung zur Überlieferung der Schriften des Theophanes Chrysobalantes (sog. Theophanes Nonnus)* (Freie Universität Berlin, Byzantinisch-Neogriechisches Seminar, ΠΟΙΚΙΛΑ ΒΥΖΑΝΤΙΝΑ 7). Bonn: Dr. Rudolf Habelt, 1987.

Sprengel 1829: Kurt Sprengel (ed.), *Pedanii Dioscoridis Anazarbei De materia medica ad fidem codicum manuscriptorum, editionis aldinae principis usquequaque neglectae, et interpretum priscroum textum recnesuit, varias addidit lectiones, interpretationem emendavit, commentario illustravit*, Tomus I (Medicorum graecorum opoera quae exstant 1). Lipsiae: Cnobloch, 1829.

Thorndike and Kibre 1937: Lynn Thorndike, and Pearl Kibre, *A Catalogue of Incipits of Mediaeval Scientific Writings in Latin* (Mediaeval Academy of America, Publication 29). Cambridge, MA: Mediaeval Academy of America, 1937.

Thorndike and Kibre 1963: Lynn Thorndike, and Pearl Kibre, *A Catalogue of Incipits of Mediaeval Scientific Writings in Latin*. Revised and augmented edition (Mediaeval Academy of America, Publication 29). Cambridge, MA: Mediaeval Academy of America, 1963.

Touwaide 2009: Alain Touwaide, "Byzantine Medical Manuscripts. Towards a New Catalogue, with a Specimen for an Annotated Checklist of Manuscripts based on an Index of Diels' Catalogue", *Byzantion* 79 (2009), pp. 453–595.

Touwaide 2010: Alain Touwaide, "Codicology and Paleography", in Albrecht Classen (ed.), *Handbook of Medieval Studies. Terms, Methods, Trends*, 3 volumes. Berlin and New York, NY: Walter de Gruyter, 2010, vol. 1, pp. 266–329.

Touwaide 2016: Alain Touwaide, *A Census of Greek Medical Manuscripts. From Byzantium to the Renaissance* (Medicine in the Medieval Mediterranean 6). London and New York, NY: Routledge, 2016.

Touwaide 2018: Alain Touwaide, "Towards a Catalogue of Greek Medical Manuscripts", in Paola Degni, Paolo Eleuteri, and Marilena Maniaci (eds), *Greek Manuscript Cataloguing: Past, Present, and Future* (Bibliologia. Elementa ad librorum studia pertinentia 47). Turnhout: Brepols, 2018, pp. 111–118.

Tselikas 1995: Ἀγαμέμνων Τσελίκας, "Τὰ ἑλληνικὰ γιατροσόφια: μιὰ περιφρονημένη κατηγορία χειρογράφων", in Thanasis Diamantopoulos (ed.), Ιατρικά Βυζάντινα χειρόγραφα. Αθήνα: Δόμος, 1995, pp. 57–69.

Tselikas 2014: Ἀγαμέμνων Τσελίκας, "Δύο συναγωγὲς ἰατρικῶν λέξεων καὶ ἰατρικὲς συνταγὲς ἀπὸ τὸν ἰατροσοφικὸ κώδικα Παναγίου Τάφου 339 τοῦ Πατριαρχείου Ἱρουσολύμων", in *Εὔκρατον-Πρακτικά Επιστημονικής Συνάντησης προς τιμήν του κ. Γεωργίου Ν. Αντονακοπούλου ομότιμου καθηγητού της Ιατρικής Σχολής του Πανεπιστημίου Θεσσαλίας. Λάρισσα 10 Μαΐου 2014, Αμφι-*

θέατρο Δημοσίας Κεντρικής Βιβλιοθήκης Λάρισσας «Κωνσταντίνος Κούμας». Λάρισσα: Δημοσίας Κεντρικής Βιβλιοθήκης Λάρισσας «Κωνσταντίνος Κούμας» – Ιατρική Σχολή Πανεπιστημίου Θεσσαλίας, 2014, pp. 107–176.

Tselikas and Ilioudis 1995: Ἀγαμέμνων Τσελίκας, Γιάννης Ἠλιούδης, *Νικολάου Ἱερόπαιδος ἐξ Ἀγράφων, Πραγματεία περὶ Φυσιολογίας καὶ Παθολογίας* (Βιβλιοθήκη Νεωτέρων Ἑλληνῶν Ἰατρῶν 1). Λάρισα: Πανεπιστήμιο Θεσσαλίας, Τμῆμα Ἰατρικῆς, 1995.

Tselikas and Ilioudis 1997: Ἀγαμέμνων Τσελίκας, Γιάννης Ἠλιούδης, *Νικολάου Ἱερόπαιδος ἐξ Ἀγράφων, Ἐκδόσεις μερικαὶ εἰς ἀρχάριον ἰατρόν* (Βιβλιοθήκη Νεωτέρων Ἑλληνῶν Ἰατρῶν 2). Λάρισα: Πανεπιστήμιο Θεσσαλίας, Τμῆμα Ἰατρικῆς, 1997.

Turyn 1932: Aleksander Turyn, *De Codicibus Pindaricis* (Polska Akademja Umiejętności: Archiwum Filologiczne 11). Cracoviae: Academia Polonae Litterarum, 1932.

Turyn 1943: Aleksander Turyn, *The Manuscript Tradition of the Tragedies of Aeschylus*. New York, NY: Polish Institute of Arts and Sciences in America, 1943.

Turyn 1952: Alexander Turyn, *Studies in the Manuscript Tradition of the Tragedies of Sophocles* (Illinois Studies in Language and Literature 36, 1–2.). Urbana, IL: University of Illinois Press, 1952.

Turyn 1957: Alexander Turyn, *The Byzantine Manuscript Tradition of the Tragedies of Euripides* (Illinois Studies in Language and Literature 43). Urbana, IL: University of Illinois Press, 1957.

Ullmann 1970: Manfred Ullmann, *Die Medizin im Islam* (Handbuch der Orientalistik, Erste Abteilung: Der nahe und der mittlere Osten, Ergänzungsband VI, 1. Abschnitt). Leiden and Köln: Brill, 1970.

Verner 1966: Mathilde Verner "Johann Albert Fabricius, Eighteenth-Century Scholar and Bibliographer", *The Papers of the Bibliographical Society of America* 60 (3) (1966), pp. 281–326.

Voigts and Kurtz 2004: Linda Ersham Voigts, and Patricia Deery Kurtz, *Electronic Thorndike Kibre (eTK) and Electronic Voigts Kurtz (eVK)*. CD Rom publication, release 20 August 2004.

Vollmer 1916: Fridericus Vollmer, *Quinti Sereni Liber medicinalis*. Edidit – (Corpus Medicorum Latinorum II 3). Lipsiae et Berolini: B. G. Teubner, 1916.

Wellmann 1908: Max Wellmann (ed.), *Philumeni de venenatis animalibus eorumque remediis ex codice vaticano* primum edidit (Corpus Medicorum Graecorum X 1, 1). Lipsiae et Berolini: B. G. Teubner, 1908.

Wenkebach 1934: Ernst Wenkebach (ed.), *Galeni, In Hippocratis epidemiarum librum I commentarii III*; Franz Pfarr (Germ. transl.), *Galeni, In Hippocratis epidemiarum librum II commentarii V* (Corpus Medicorum Graecorum V 10, 1). Lipsiae et Berolini: B. G. Teubner, 1934.

Wenkebach 1936: Ernst Wenkebach (ed.), *Galeni, In Hippocratis epidemiarum librum IIII commentarii III* (Corpus Medicorum Graecorum V 10, 2. 1). Lipsiae et Berolini: B. G. Teubner, 1936.

Wilson 1987: Nigel G. Wilson, "Aspects of the Transmission of Galen", in Guglielmo Cavallo (ed.), *Le strade del testo* (Studi e commenti 5). Bari: Adriatica Editrice, 1987, pp. 45–64.

Zipser 2009: Barbara Zipser (ed.), *John the Physician's Therapeutics. A Medical Handbook in Vernacular Greek* (Studies in Ancient Medicine 37). Leiden: Brill, 2009.

Acknowledgements

This work is the result of decades of intensive activity in libraries, research centers, universities, and other institutions throughout the world, which have all provided resources, access to collections, expertise and guidance and, most simply, a home. I am pleased to thank all of them and their staff, even though I cannot enumerate them here. In very recent years, the work has benefitted from the active support of De Gruyter, particularly the Senior Editor for Classical Studies Dr. Serena Pirrotta and her team, especially Marco Acquafredda, and De Gruyter computer and technical units in the persons of Anne Hiller and Florian Ruppenstein who have provided much needed assistance. Going slightly back in time, Patricia Kellogg has been an efficient research assistant and Cheyenne Moore has checked the accuracy of my index of Diels against the original. Since its foundation in 2007 the *Institute for the Preservation of Medical Traditions* has hosted the programme. In the very last phase, Marisa Gomez has checked with great linguistic talent the correctness of the introduction to the several parts of the work. More than anyone else, Emanuela Appetiti has accompanied me through multiple peregrinations of all kinds of which this work may give only an imperfect idea. I cannot conclude without remembering Joseph A. M. Sonderkamp with whom I discussed the project of a *New Diels* and a catalogue of Greek medical manuscripts as early as 1983 in Berlin and then in 1987 at Louvain-la-Neuve. We had defined a cooperative programme and had started implementing it when the sinister *Moira* decided shortly after that we would not fully realize it in collaboration.

Index of Manuscripts
Diels' Location and Shelfmark

Notes for consultation

This index lists all the manuscripts with texts by other physicians than Hippocrates and Galen mentioned in Diels. The identifications exactly reproduce the data provided in Diels, the majority of which comprise the following three or four components: city (German form), library (mostly in the original language, often in an abbreviated form, and in their form as in Diels' time), collection (when appropriate), and one or more shelfmarks or references to an earlier work. In some cases, the name of the library is not explicitly mentioned; it can be identified through the list of catalogues in Diels' bibliography. The index references the page number(s) where each item appears in the present volume.

This index is preceded by a **Finding Aid** which lists the city, library and collection names in alphabetical order with reference to the present index, and two lists: one with the names as in Diels (sometimes including transliteration into the Latin alphabet for Greek names) and the other with their current standard English form.

Finding Aid
City and Library names

1. Names according to Diels

2. Standard English names

Index of Manuscripts

Index of Manuscripts
Current location and shelfmark

Notes for consultation

This index lists all the Greek manuscripts with texts by other physicians than Hippocrates and Galen mentioned in Diels that have been preserved and identified since[1]. Their designation comprises their current location and shelfmark, with the following three or four components: city, library, collection (when appropriate), and shelfmark. All names are in the original language and alphabet, followed by their transliteration into Latin alphabet and translation into English for those in the original Russian and Armenian alphabet and form. Each entry of the index references the page number(s) in this volume where the manuscripts appear.

Since the manuscripts contained in the catalogue in this volume are identified as they are in Diels, consultation of the catalogue on the basis of this index might be problematic because current designations do not always match Diels' designations. In Diels, indeed, cities are identified by their German names, libraries are often designated in an abbreviated form, collection names are abbreviated or may not reflect actual names, and shelfmarks are sometimes insufficient or inexact, or even include earlier ones. Additionally, changes have occurred since Diels' time in the location of some collections and several manuscripts, in the names of some libraries and, also, in the shelfmarks (and even in the shelfmark system) of several libraries. Diels' identifiers are reproduced between parentheses after the page number referring to the mention(s) of the manuscripts in the catalogue contained in this volume. In the catalogue itself, both designations of manuscripts are included when appropriate, followed by the current one (as listed in the present index).

This index is preceded by a **Finding Aid** which provides the current city, library, and collection names in alphabetical order with reference to the present index. All names are in the original language and alphabet.

1 This index does not include the manuscripts that have been lost or destroyed (*in toto* or *in parte*) since (e.g. some items from Dresden or Torino), the manuscripts that cannot be exactly identified on the basis of Diels' information, the papyri, and the Latin and Arabic manuscripts included among the Greek manuscripts in Diels. The identifications reproduce those in Touwaide 2016.

Finding Aid

City and Library names

2 Actually Μοναστική Πολιτεία Αγίου Όρους.

Index of Manuscripts

[3] Actually Μοναστική Πολιτεία Αγίου Όρους.

Φ. III. 12: 38
X. I. 11: 38
X. II. 2: 38
X. II. 9: 38
Ψ. I. 13: 38
Ψ. III. 7: 39
Ψ. IV. 14: 39
Ω. I. 8: 39

Sáros-Patak, Sárospatakai Református Kollégium Todományos Gyüjteményei, Nagykönyvtár
Kt 405: 165 (Sáros-Patak, Bibl. d. reform. Colleg.)

Toledo, Biblioteca Capitular, Catedral de Toledo
Fondo Zelada
BCT 101–15: 166 (Toledo, Bibl. del cab. de la igl. Catedr. 101, 15)

Torino, Biblioteca Nazionale Universitaria
See Turin, Bibl. Nationale (Universitaria)
B. I. 6: 166 (6 b IV 6)
C. VI. 3: 166 (287 c I 42)
C. VI. 10: 166 (156 b II 10)
C. VI. 21: 167 (C VI 21 [b VI 18])

Tübingen, Universitätsbibliothek
See Tübingen, Univ.-Bibl.
Mb 2: 166 (2)

Uppsala, Uppsala Universitet
See Upsala, Upsal. bibl. acad.
Gr
8: 167 (8 (e don. Jo. Gabr. Sparfwenf. 49)
30: 167 (30)
34: 167 (34)

Venezia, Biblioteca Nazionale Marciana
See Venedig, Bibl. National Marciana
graeci
173 (coll. 476): 168 (173)
257 (coll. 622): 168 (257)
266 (coll. 517): 169 (266)

Catalogue of Manuscripts

Notes for consultation

The catalogue that follows collects and exactly reproduces the data presented for the Greek manuscripts containing other texts that the Hippocatic and Galenic ones listed in Diels[1]. Each manuscript received an entry in which data are divided in two major parts: identification (followed by possible annotations) and contents.

Identifications of the manuscripts comprise a city and library name, a collection when appropriate, and a shelfmark. City names are mostly in German, whereas library names are either in German or in the original language (and in the Greek alphabet for several, but not all, of the libraries in Greece). The library names used by Diels do not always follow the actual form they had in Diels' time and, whatever their exactness, they are often in an abbreviated form. Collection names are either those of the libraries (often in an abbreviated form) or Latin adjectives formed on the name of the city. Shelfmarks are those used when Diels was compiled or sometimes, earlier ones, or even both. For some manuscripts, erroneous shelfmarks provided in the first two issues of Diels are corrected in the *Nachtrag* (Supplement). In some cases, Diels does not provide a shelfmark, but only a reference to a citation in an earlier catalogue or a more recent publication. For several items, all or some of these data (specifically the shelfmarks) appear between brackets in Diels (sometimes also with a question mark within the brackets) to indicate that they are reproduced from Ackermann (1791 and 1796) or Littré (1839–1861)[2]. The year or, in most cases, the century of copy of the manuscripts follows. For several manuscripts this chronological indication varies from one occurrence to another. All such divergent estimates are provided here in chronological order. In the catalogue contained in this volume, all these data form the first line of the entry devoted to each manuscript; they are printed in boldface for the purposes of easy and direct consultation. Notes about the possible untraceability and the state of preservation of some manuscripts, as well as possible corrections of shelfmark and time of copy provided in the *Nachtrag* (Supplement) are reproduced in the next line, printed in italic.

When necessary, the identification of the manuscripts is followed (on the next line) by annotations providing the correspondence between Diels' and current identi-

1 Only manuscripts that have been preserved and precisely identified are listed here. Items lost (already in Diels' time or later), destroyed (including because of the two World Wars), missing, or mentioned in Diels, but not precisely identified as per the *Census*, have been omitted. They appear, however, in the catalogue of manuscripts in tome 5.

2 See p. 2 in the 1905 issue for an explanation of the brackets.

fication of the manuscripts since several Diels identifiers do not correspond to their actual or current equivalent (from the city names in German to possible changes of shelfmarks). Correspondences (particularly of shelfmarks) that could not be established with a degree of certainty are introduced by a question mark. All correspondences reproduce those provided in the *Census of Greek Medical Manuscripts* (2016), which is referenced between parentheses after the current identification. To avoid repetition among the entries when several manuscripts appear in the same library or collection, Diels' and current names are provided only once, at the beginning of the section of the catalogue devoted to the library or the collection.

A special case is that of the manuscripts listed in Diels under different shelfmarks or with a shelfmark between brackets. Each distinct shelfmark in Diels has received an entry. However, all such entries include a reference to the manuscripts they refer to and, conversely, they are referred to in the entry of the manuscripts they are related to. These cross-references follow the identification of the manuscripts (Diel's and current). Shelfmarks (or other identifiers) referred to are printed in boldface to allow for easy cross-referencing.

The second and most substantial part of each entry details the contents of the manuscripts. All the texts included in Diels (and only those) are listed here in the same order as in the manuscripts, with the following four descriptors: the folios where they appear or their sequential number in the manuscripts (in both cases between parentheses), the author's name, the title of the work (in italic), and any possible notes of commentary between parentheses (*incipit*, lacunae, *desinit*, source, comparison with other texts, or any other philological or textual peculiarity as identified in Diels, sometimes with the name of Diels' collaborator who provided the information). References to other manuscripts (sometimes without precise shelfmark in Diels) have been made explicit (via shelfmark between brackets) to allow for cross-referencing. The asterisk that follows the title of some works in Diels to indicate a fragmentary text has been replaced by the explicit mention *Frgm*. References to the parts and pages of Diels' catalogue, and mentions of collations made or owned by Diels' collaborators have been omitted, as have also been some notes historico-critical in nature.

Athen, Βιβλ. τῆς Βουλῆς
Now Αθήνα, Βιβλιοθήκη της Βουλής των Ελλήνων

Athen, Βιβλ. τῆς Βουλῆς, 43; s. XIII.

Meletius monachus: (f. 122) *De natura hominis.*

Athen, Βιβλ. τῆς Βουλῆς, 68; s. XVIII.

Asclepiades, Dioscurides: (f. 212) *Praecepta salubria* (Asclep. et Dioscr. ὑγιεινὰ παραγγέλματα. Inc. Μεταδιδόασθαι τὴν τροφὴν ἐξορμήσας ἀταμιεύτως).
Hippokrates, Paulus Aegineta, Paulus Nicaeensis: (f. 220) *De morbis* (Exc. varia περὶ παθῶν ex Hipp., Gal., Paulo Nic., Paulo Aeg.).

Athen, Nationalbibl.
Αθήνα, Εθνική Βιβλιοθήκη της Ελλάδος ΕΒΕ

Athen, Nationalbibl., 375; s. XIII.

Nemesius Emesenus: (nr 11) *De natura hominis.*

Athen, Nationalbibl., 433 (132); s. XII.
= 433 (*Census*: 11, nr [0007]).

Gregorius Nyssenus: (nr 2) *De hominis opificio* (Κεφάλαια λ').

Athen, Nationalbibl., 447 (146); s. XVI.
= 447 (*Census*: 11, nr [0008]).

Nemesius Emesenus: (nr 16) *De natura hominis.*

Athen, Nationalbibl., 1180; s. XVIII.

Hermes Trismegistus: (nr 1) *Ad Asclepium liber generalis.*

Athen, Nationalbibl., 1236; s. XVIII.

Diocles: *Ad Antigonum regem epistula de tuenda valetitudine.*

Athen, Nationalbibl., 1478.

Nicolaus Myrepsus: *De compositione medicamentorum, alphabetice* (*vgl.* Krumbacher, Byz. Litt.[2] 617f. »Phillipps. 1583 [below p. 22] hat mit diesem Werke nichts zu tun, muß also fort; ebenso muß fort Parisin. 2315 [below p. 131]; f. 276. Da steht nur ἑρμενία νικολάου, περὶ ἐμπλάστρου πάνυ ὠφέλιμον. Hinzuzufügen wäre noch [nach Foerster p. 31] aus der Rhädestosbibliothek: νικολάου τοῦ μυρεψικοῦ ἰατρικόν. Und endlich ist zu erwähnen, daß es eine lateinische Übersetzung des Werkes gibt, Ingolst. 1549, vom Tübinger Leonhard Fuchs. Die Handschrift, die er benutzt hat, scheint verloren. Die Übersetzung ist bei Stephanus und sonst öfter wieder gedruckt.« Treu).

Athen, Nationalbibl., 1479; s. XIX.

Galenos, Paulus Aegineta, Dioscurides: *Excerpta/Iatrosophia* (Ἰατροσόφιον ἀπηνθισμένον ἀπὸ Γαλ., Παύλου τοῦ Αἰγ. ... καὶ Δ.).

Athen, Nationalbibl., 1480; s. XIX.

Dioscurides: *Opera varia* (Δ. τὰ ἅπαντα εἰς τὸ κατὰ στοιχεῖον μετακοσμηθέντα ὑπὸ Ἀντωνίου Ποθητοῦ τοῦ Ναξίου).

Athen, Nationalbibl., 1481; s. XVI.

Neophytus Prodromenus: (nr 1) *De dentium doloribus.*
Ioannes Episcopus Prisdianensis: (nr 3) *Collectanea de urinis.*

Athen, Nationalbibl., 1494; s. XVIII.

Theophilus: (nr 2) *De alvi excrementis.*

Athen, Nationalbibl., 1506; s. XIX.

Meletius monachus: *Excerpta varia* (Μελετίου ἰατροσόφιον).

Athos, Βιβλ. Μον. Βατοπεδίου
Now Ἅγιον Ὄρος, Ιερά Μονή Βατοπεδίου

Athos, Βιβλ. Μον. Βατοπεδίου, A 29; s. –; XIV.
Now Ἅγιον Ὄρος, Ιερά Μονή Βατοπεδίου, 29 (*Census*: 16, nr [0027]).

Aëtius Amidenus: *Iatricorum libri XVI* (Es fehlen B. V c. 137–143, VI und Schluß von XVI).

Athos, Βιβλ. Μον. Διονυσίου
Now Άγιον Όρος, Ιερά Μονή Διονυσίου

Athos, Βιβλ. Μον. Διονυσίου, 3748. 214; s. XV.
Now 263 (*Census*: 16, nr [0029]).

Gregorius Nyssenus: (nr 1) *De hominis opificio* (Κεφ. λ').
Gregorius Theologus: (nr 2) *De compositione et distinctione corporis humani* (Ποιήματα ... ιγ'. Περὶ φύσεως ἀνθρωπίνης).

Athos, Βιβλ. Μον. Διονυσίου, 3766. 232; s. XVII.
Now 474.

Epiphanius: (nr 25) *Physiologus*.

Athos, Βιβλ. Μον. Διονυσίου, 3778. 244; s. XVII.
Now 283.

Epiphanius: (nr 2) *Physiologus* (Frgm.).

Athos, Βιβλ. Μον. Διονυσίου, 3799. 265; s. XV.
Now 297 (*Census*: 17, nr [0033]).

Nemesius Emesenus: (nr 2) *De natura hominis*.

Athos, Βιβλ. Μον. Διονυσίου, 3808. 274; s. XVI.
Now 168 (*Census*: 17, nr [0034]).

Gregorius Nyssenus: (f. 333) *De hominis opificio* (Π. φύσεως ἀνθρώπου).

Athos, Βιβλ. Μον. Διονυσίου, 3881. 347; s. XVI.
Now 402 (*Census*: 17, nr [0035]).

Lucas: (f. 195) *Compositio salsi intinctus*.

Athos, Βιβλ. Μον. Διονυσίου, 3897. 363; s. XVIII.
Now 206.

Epiphanius: (nr 7) *Physiologus* (Frgm.).

Athos, Βιβλ. Μον. Ἰβήρων
Now Άγιον Όρος, Ιερά Μονή Ιβήρων

Athos, Βιβλ. Μον. Ἰβήρων, 151; s. XV.
= 151 (4271) (*Census*: 18, nr [0041]).
See also **4271. 151** below.

Ioannes Zacharias Actuarius: *De methodo medendi libri VI* (Liber V).

Athos, Βιβλ. Μον. Ἰβήρων, 4212. 92; s. XVI.
= 92 (4212) (*Census*: 10, nr [0042]).

Epiphanius: (f. 28. 31) *De mensuris et ponderibus.*

Athos, Βιβλ. Μον. Ἰβήρων, 4271. 151; s. XV.
Same as **151** above (*Census*: 19, nr [0043]).
= 151 (4271).

Logadius: *Excerpta* (Ἱερά. Inc. Κολοκυντίδι ἐτεριώνην ὀγκίας κ' σκίλλης ὀπτῆς).
Paulus Aegineta: (f. 8^{v}) *De succedaneis, ex Galeno.*
Nicomedes Iatrosophista: (f. 11) *Lexicon* (Inc. Ἀκτὶς ἡ κουφοξυλέα. Expl. Ὤνια τὰ ἐν ταῖς δρύαις [?] ζῷα. ὑποσταθμὴ ἐλαίου τρυγαῖα).
Gregorius Theologus: (f. 70 B) *Alatium.*
Paulus Aegineta: (f. 125) *De succedaneis, ex Galeno.*
Ocianus: (f. 184) *De compositione medicamentorum.*
Andreiomenus: (f. 228) *Notae medicae.*

Athos, Βιβλ. Μον. Ἰβήρων, 4272. 152; s. XVI.
= 152 (4272) (*Census*: 19, nr [0044]).

Epiphanius: (f. 40) *Physiologus.*

Athos, Βιβλ. Μον. Ἰβήρων, 4301. 181; s. XVI.
= 181 (4301) (*Census*: 19, nr [0048]).

Adamantius: (f. 2) *De palpitionibus.*

Athos, Βιβλ. Μον. Ἰβήρων, 4302. 181; s. XVI.
Same as **4302. 182** below (*Census*: 19, nr [0049]).
= 182 (4302).

Oribasius: (f. 29 B–145) *Excerpta varia* (Ἰατροσόφιον κατ' ἀλφάβητον).
Diocles: (f. 158) *Ad Antigonum regem epistula de tuenda valetudine.*
Eutecnius: (f. 167) *Paraphrasis in Nicandri Alexipharmaca.*

Athos, Βιβλ. Μον. Ἰβήρων, 4302. 182; s. XVI.
= 182 (4302) (*Census*: 19, nr [0050]).
See also **4302. 181** above.

Salomo: (f. 7) *Praecepta* (»Praecepta quorum nonnulla secundum Salomonicum«).

Athos, Βιβλ. Μον. Ἰβήρων, 4310. 190; s. XIII.
= 190 (4310) (*Census*: 20, nr [0053]).

Epiphanius: (nr 1) *Physiologus*.

Athos, Βιβλ. Μον. Ἰβήρων, 4325. 205; s. XVII.
= 205 (4325) (*Census*: 20, nr [0054]).

Epiphanius: (f. 153) *Physiologus*.

Athos, Βιβλ. Μον. Ἰβήρων, 4336. 216; s. XV.
= 216 (4336) (*Census*: 20, nr [0056]).

Eutecnius: *Paraphrasis in Oppiani Halieutica* (Inc. Αἱ ῥαφίδες τῷ λίνῳ πρὸς τὸν αἰγιαλόν).
Dioscurides: (f. 1) *De materia medica*.

Athos, Βιβλ. Μον. Ἰβήρων, 4337. 217; s. XVI.
= 217 (4337) (*Census*: 20, nr [0057]).

Dioscurides:
(f. 10) *De facile parabilibus tam simplicibus quam compositis medicamentis libri II*.
(f. 51 B) *Excerpta* (Ἑρμηνεία τοῦ Δ. περὶ τοῦ καρωφάλου [sic] καὶ ἄλλων ἑτέρων).

Athos, Βιβλ. Μον. Ἰβήρων, 4340. 220; s. XVII.
= 220 (4340) (*Census*: 21, nr [0060]).

Aëtius Amidenus: *Excerpta varia* (Π. φλεβοτομίας).

Athos, Βιβλ. Μον. Ἰβήρων, 4436. 316; s. XV.
= 316 (4436) (*Census*: 21, nr [0061]).

Oribasius:
(f. 102) *Conspectus ad Eustathium filium. Libri II* (Frgm. Ὅσα θερμαίνει μετρίως).
(f. 102) *Ad Eunapium de parabilibus medicamentis. Libri IV* (Frgm.).

Paulus Aegineta:
(f. 134 B) *Epitomae medicae libri septem* (Lib. I Διόρθωσις τῶν θερμῶν δυσκρασίων).
(f. 136 A) *Epitomae medicae libri septem* (Ἴασις τῶν ξηρῶν δυσκρασίων κτλ.).

Athos, Βιβλ. Μον. Ἰβήρων, 4450. 330; s. XVIII.
= 330 (4450) (*Census*: 21, nr [0062]).

Epiphanius: (nr 11) *Physiologus* (Π. φύσεως ἑκάστου).

Athos, Βιβλ. Μον. Ἰβήρων, 4468. 348; s. XVI.
= 348 (4468) (*Census*: 21, nr [0064]).

Epiphanius: (nr 10) *Physiologus*.

Athos, Βιβλ. Μον. Ἰβήρων, 4497. 377; s. XIV.
= 377 (4497) (*Census*: 21, nr [0065]).

Epiphanius: (f. 106) *Physiologus*.

Athos, Βιβλ. Μον. Ἰβήρων, 4655. 535; s. XVI.
= 535 (4655) (*Census*: 21, nr [0068]).

Galenos, Hippokrates, Meletius monachus: *Iatrosophia/excerpta varia* (Ἰατροσόφη ἐκλελεγμένον ὑπὸ ... Γαλ. Ἱππ. καὶ Μελ. καὶ ἄλλων δοκίμων ἰατρῶν. Cap. 1. Ὅτι ὁ κόσμος ὑπὸ τεσσάρων στοιχείων).

Athos, Βιβλ. Μον. Ἰβήρων, 4720. 600; s. XVII.
= 600 (4720) (*Census*: 21, nr [0070]).

Epiphanius: (nr 21) *Physiologus*.

Athos, Βιβλ. Μον. Ἰβήρων, 4788. 668; s. XVIII.
= 668 (4788) (*Census*: 22, nr [0071]).

Epiphanius: (nr 28) *Physiologus* (Frgm.).

Athos, Βιβλ. Μον. Ἰβήρων, 4799. 679; s. XVIII.
= 679 (4799) (*Census*: 22, nr [0073]).

Epiphanius: (nr 4) *Physiologus*.

Athos, Βιβλ. Μον. Ἰβήρων, 4815. 695; s. XVI.
= 695 (4815) (*Census*: 22, nr [0074]).

Epiphanius: (nr 2) *Physiologus*.

Athos, Βιβλ. Μον. Ἰβήρων, 4871. 751; s. XVII.
= 751 (4871) (*Census*: 22, nr [0075]).

Epiphanius: (nr 53) *De mensuris et ponderibus*.

Athos, Βιβλ. Μον. Ἰβήρων, 4925. 805; s. XVII.
= 805 (4925) (*Census*: 22, nr [0076]).

Epiphanius: (f. 80) *Physiologus*.

Athos, Βιβλ. Μον. Κουτλουμουσίου
Now Άγιον Όρος, Ιερά Μονή Κουτλουμουσίου

Athos, Βιβλ. Μον. Κουτλουμουσίου, 3260. 2; s. XVI.
= 187 (3260) (*Census*: 22–23, nr [0079]).

Epiphanius: (nr 2) *Physiologus*.

Athos, Βιβλ. Μον. Κουτλουμουσίου, 3321. 248; s. XVII.
= 248 (3321) (*Census*: 23, nr [0080]).

Dioscurides: *Excerpta* (Δ. περὶ ἁπλῶν βοηθημάτων ἐν βίβλῳ ἰατρικῇ Νικολάου Ἱερόπαιδος).
Oribasius: *Excerpta varia*.

Athos, Βιβλ. Μον. Λαύρας
Now Άγιον Όρος, Ιερά Μονή Μεγίστης Λαύρας

Athos, Βιβλ. Μον. Λαύρας, –; s. XII.
= Ω 75 (*Census*: 23–24, nr [0082]).

Dioscurides:
(f. 6) *De mensuris et ponderibus*.
(f. 9) *De materia medica* (alphab.).
(f. 218) *De venenis eorumque praecautione et medicatione* (Inscr. Περὶ τῆς τῶν ὠφελεῖν ἢ βλάπτειν δυναμένων φαρμάκων ἐνεργείας).
(f. 227) *De iis, quae virus eiaculantur, animalibus libellus, in quo et de rabioso cane*.
Eutecnius:
(f. 242) *Paraphrasis in Nicandri Theriaca*.
(f. 260) *Paraphrasis in Nicandri Alexipharmaca*.

(f. 273) *Paraphrasis in Oppiani Halieutica* (Inc. *wie im* cod. Ἰβήρων [4336. 216] [see p. 9]. Expl. τοῖς ἰχθύσι οἱ θηραταί).
(f. 285) *Paraphrasis in Dionysii Ixeutica* (Inscriptionis expers).

Athos, Βιβλ. Μον. Λαύρας, *Ausser* Ω 70 *und* 72 *noch 4 weitere Hdss. bei* Costomiris Rev. des ét. gr. III [1890] p. 166 *und* 127.
= Ω 63, Ω 64, Ω 65, Ω 66 (*Census*: 24–25, nos [0083], [0084], [0085], [0086], respectively).

Aëtius Amidenus: *Libri medicinales.*

Athos, Βιβλ. Μον. Λαύρας, Ω 69; s. –.

Ioannes Zacharias Actuarius: *Tractatus de urinis, qui ex Avicenna translatus dicitur in graecam linguam a Christodulo, in ordinem redactus ab Actuario Zacharia.*

Athos, Βιβλ. Μον. Λαύρας, Ω 70, –; a. ,ϛϡμε′ (= 1437).

Aëtius Amidenus: *Iatricorum libri XVI.*

Athos, Βιβλ. Μον. Λαύρας, Ω 72; s. –; XIV.

Aëtius Amidenus: *Iatricorum libri XVI.*

Athos, Βιβλ. Μον. Παντελεήμονος
Now Άγιον Όρος, Ιερά Μονή Παντελεήμονος

Athos, Βιβλ. Μον. Παντελεήμονος, 5752. 245; s. XVII.
= 245 (5752) (*Census*: 25, nr [0091]).

Epiphanius: (nr 5) *Physiologus.*

Athos, Βιβλ. Μον. Παντελεήμονος, 5768. 261; s. XVIII.
= 261 (5768) (*Census*: 25, nr [0092]).

Meletius monachus: *Excerpta varia* (Τοῦ πανιερωτάτου καὶ λογιωτάτου μητροπολίτου Ναυπάκτου καὶ Ἄρτης κυρίου, κυρίου Μελετίου, Εἰσαγώγη διαφόρων ἀκουσμάτων καὶ ἰατρικῶν).

Athos, Βιβλ. Μον. Παντελεήμονος, 5769. 262; s. XVIII.
= 262 (5769) (*Census*: 25, nr [0093]).

Meletius monachus, Hippokrates, Galenos, Paulus Aegineta: (f. 15 [15 A]) *Excerpta varia* (Ἰατροσόφιον ἐκλελεγμένον ὑπὸ πολλῶν ἰατρικῶν βιβλ. Γαλ. Ἱππ. Μελ. καὶ Παύλ. τοῦ Αἰγ. συγγραφὲν δὲ παρὰ Κοσμᾶ ἱερομονάχου τοῦ Μακεδόνος).

Athos, Βιβλ. Μον. Παντελεήμονος, 6351. 844; s. XVIII.
= 844 (6351) (*Census*: 26, nr [0096]).

Salomo: (f. 42) *Praecepta* (Σολομωνικὴ μετὰ προγνωστικῶν).

Athos, Βιβλ. Μον. Παντελεήμονος, 6372. 865; s. XIX.
= 865 (6372) (*Census*: 26, nr [0097]).

Meletius monachus: (f. 205 B) *Excerpta varia* (Ἀποσημειώσεις τινὲς ψυχωφελεῖς. *Darunter* Τοῦ ἁγίου Μελετίου τοῦ ὁμολογητοῦ Περὶ διαίτης ὁλικῶς).

Athos, Βιβλ. Μον. Ξηροποτάμου
Now Άγιον Όρος, Ιερά Μονή Ξηροποτάμου

Athos, Βιβλ. Μον. Ξηροποτάμου, 2432. 99; s. XVII.
= 99 (2432) (*Census*: 26, nr [0099]).

Dioscurides: *Excerpta* (Διαθήκη τῶν τριῶν ἰατρῶν Γαλ. Ἱππ. καὶ Δ.).

Athos, Σταυρονικήτα
Now Άγιον Όρος, Ιερά Μονή Σταυρονικήτα

Athos, Σταυρονικήτα, 951. 86; s. XVII.
Άγιον Όρος, Ιερά Μονή Σταυρονικήτα, 86 (951) (*Census*: 26, nr [0101]).

Epiphanius: (nr 5) *Physiologus*.

Athos, Ξενοφῶντος
Now Ἅγιον Ὄρος, Ιερά Μονή Ξενοφῶντος

Athos, Ξενοφῶντος, 739. 37; s. XVIII.
Ἅγιον Ὄρος, Ιερά Μονή Ξενοφῶντος, 37 (739) (*Census*: 26, nr [0102]).

Gregorius Nyssenus: *De hominis opificio* (Π. ἀνθρώπου κεφ. λ).

Basel

Basel, Bibl. univ., F VI 46; s. XVI.
Now Öffentliche Bibliothek der Universität Basel, Mscr F VI 46 (*Census*: 27, nr [0103]).

Paulus Aegineta: (f. 9) *Epitomae medicae libri septem* (L. VI 15. 16).

Berlin, Königl. Bibl.
Now Staatsbibliothek zu Berlin – Preussischer Kulturbesitz SBB-PKB

Berlin, Königl. Bibl., 4° 2 (301); s. XVII.
Now Ms. graec. quart. 2 (*Census*: 27, nr [0106]).

Marcellus Sidetes: (f. 37ᵛ) *Medicina ex piscibus.*

Berlin, Königl. Bibl., 4° 5 (304); s. XV–XVI.
Now Kraków, Biblioteka Jagiellońska, quarto 5 (*Census*: 28, nr [0107], 103).

Epiphanius: (f. 70ᵛ) *De duodecim gemmis panno sacerdotis infibulatis.*
Meletius monachus: (f. 53ᵛ) *De natura hominis* (Διαθήκη τῶν τριῶν ἰατρῶν Γαλην. Ἱππ. καὶ Μελετίου ... περὶ τῆς τοῦ ἀνθρώπου κατασκευῆς καὶ πῶς δεῖ διεξιέναι τὸν καιρόν).

Berlin, Königl. Bibl., qu. 46 (348); s. XVI.
Now Kraków, Biblioteka Jagiellońska, quarto 46 (*Census*: 33, nr [0153], 103).

Meletius monachus: *Excerpta varia*: ρνθ' (Στίχοι πάνυ ὠφέλιμοι Μελετίου) *und* ρξ' (Περὶ τοῦ παραγενομένου εἰς ἰατρίαν ἀδελφοῦ).

Berlin, Königl. Bibl., fol. 7 (247); s. XVI.
Now Kraków, Biblioteka Jagiellońska, folio 7 (*Census*: 28, nr [0109], 103).

Ioannes Zacharias Actuarius: (f. 1) *De urinis libri VII.*

Berlin, Königl. Bibl., fol. 35 (271); s. IX.
= Ms. graec. fol. 35.

Oribasius: *Medicae collectiones ad Iulianum* (? Frgm. Inc. προσήσθαιτο · πολλοῖς γοῦν καὶ μόνον ἐξήρκεσεν = L. VII 26, 167; Dbg.-Buss. II p. 134, 7. Expl. πρῶτον μὲν τὸ δύσεργον καὶ τοῦτο = ibid. 26, 179; Dbg.-Buss. p. 138, 5. 6).

Berlin, Königl. Bibl., fol. 37.
Now Kraków, Biblioteka Jagiellońska, folio 37 (*Census*: 28, nr [0111], 103).
See also **fol. 37 (273)** below.

Aëtius Amidenus: (f. 1) *Iatricorum libri XVI* (*Nach Zervos Apogr. des Parisin. 2191* [below p. 118]).

Berlin, Königl. Bibl., fol. 37 (273); s. XVI.
Same as **fol. 37** above.
Now Kraków, Biblioteka Jagiellońska, folio 37 (*Census*: 28, nr [0112], 103).

Aëtius Amidenus: (f. 1) *Iatricorum libri XVI.*
Africanus: (f. 501v) *De ponderibus et mensuris.*

Berlin, Königl. Bibl., fol. 38; a. 1817.
= Ms. graec. fol. 38 (*Census*: 28, nr [0113]).
See also **fol. 38 (274)** below.

Aëtius Amidenus: (f. 1) *Iatricorum libri XVI.*

Berlin, Königl. Bibl., fol. 38 (274); s. –.
Same as **fol. 38** above.
= Ms. graec. fol. 38 (*Census*: 28, nr [0114]).

Aëtius Amidenus: (f 1) *Iatricorum libri XVI* (L. IX–XVI. Apogr. cod. olim Boerhaaviani, nunc Lipsiensis).

Berlin, Königl. Bibl., fol. 39 (275); s. –, XVIII–XIX, XIX.
= Ms. graec. fol. 39 (*Census*: 28, nr [0115]).

Aëtius Amidenus: *Excerpta varia* (De alimentorum facultatibus, *Abschrift des Parisin. 1883* [p. 111]. – *Verzeichnis der Hdss. des A. in d. Vaticana*).
Alexander Aphrodisiensis: *Excerpta varia* (*Collationen kleinerer Stücke*).
Alexander Trallianus: *Excerpta varia* (*Varianten in einer Ausg. des Alex. Trall. von Gampylius in der Bibl. der Minerva zu Rom*).
Antyllus: *Excerpta varia* (*Coll. kleinerer Stücke*).
Archigenes: *Excerpta varia* (*Coll. kleinerer Stücke*).

Aretaeus:

De causis et signis acutorum morborum libri II.
De causis et signis diuturnorum morborum libri II.
De curatione acutorum morborum libri II.
De curatione diuturnorum morborum libri II (*Varianten aus* Vatic. 286 [below p. 156]. *Probecoll. von Hdss. der* Marciana).

Asclepiades: *Excerpta varia* (*Collationen kleinerer Stücke*).

Cassius iatrosophistes: *Quaestiones medicae et problemata physica* (»Abschrift von Cassius ἰατρ. ἀπ. κ. πρ. φυσ. von der Hand Bernards mit Anmerkungen und zum Teil mit lat. Übs. von demselben«).

Dioscurides: *Excerpta* (»Probecollat. von Hdss. des D. in der Marciana«).

Erotianus: *Vocum Hippocraticarum conlectio* (*Coll. vatikanischer Hdss.*).

Oribasius: *Excerpta varia* (»*Collationen kleinerer Stücke*«).

Paulus Aegineta: *Excerpta varia* (»Probecollation von P. Aeg. περὶ διαφορᾶς καὶ αἰτίας νοσημάτων nach d. Hds. des Beatus Rhenanus, verglichen mit der Baseler Ausgabe durch Schneider«).

Rufus: *Excerpta varia* (*Coll. kleinerer Stücke*).

Ioannes Zacharias Actuarius: *De methodo medendi libri VI* (»Abschr. von Buch 1. 2 von der Hand Schneiders«).

Berlin, Königl. Bibl., Phillipps.
Now Berlin, Staatsbibliothek zu Berlin – Preussischer Kulturbesitz
SBB-PKB, Ms. Phill.

Berlin, Königl. Bibl., Phillipps. 1432; s. XVI.
= Ms. Phill. 1432 (*Census*: 29, nr [0117]).

Gregorius Nyssenus: (f. 1) *De hominis opificio.*

Berlin, Königl. Bibl., Phillipps. 1524 (ol. Meerm. 214); s. XV, XVI.
= Ms. Phill. 1524 (*Census*: 29, nr [0120]).

Theophilus:

(f. 1) *Commentarius in Hippocratis aphorismos* (Inc. κείμενον · ὁ βίος βραχύς. Expl. ὅθεν ἡ ἔκλυσις γίνεται. »Codex verbis ab editione discrepat nec totum commentarium continet«).

(f. 36) *De urinis* (Inc. Κατὰ πόσας αἰτίας γίνεται ἡ ἀπεψία. Expl. καὶ τοῦτο εἰπὼν παρέλιπε).

Berlin, Königl. Bibl., Phillipps. 1525 (ol. Meerm. 215); s. XVI.
= Ms. Phill. 1525 (*Census*: 29, nr [0121]).

Palladius: (f. 1) *Scholia in Hippocratis de popularibus morbis librum sextum, sectiones VIII.*

Berlin, Königl. Bibl., Phillipps. 1527 (ol. Meerm. 217); s. XVI.
= Ms. Phill. 1527 (*Census*: 29, nr [0123]).

Theophilus: (f. 3) *De hominis fabrica Libri V* (lacunos. Expl. τὸ δὲ σχῆμα).
Gregorius Nyssenus: (f. 66^{v}) *Oratio adversus astronomos* (Frgm. Inc. Ὥσπερ οἱ ἰχθύες. Expl. ἕως ἑσπέρας).
Philo, Herennius: (f. 68^{v}) *De aetatibus hominis.*

Berlin, Königl. Bibl., Phillipps. 1528; s. XVI.
= Ms. Phill. 1528 (*Census*: 30, nr [0124]).

Ioannes Zacharias Actuarius: *De methodo medendi libri VI* (Liber VI).

Berlin, Königl. Bibl., Phillipps. 1529 (ol. Meerm. 220); s. XVI.
= Ms. Phill. 1529 (*Census*: 30, nr [0125]).

Stephanus Ἀρχιατρὸς τῶν Μαγγάνων: (f. 191^{v}) *Excerpta* (Κολλύριον ὀφθαλμικὸν παρὰ Στεφάνου ἰατροῦ τοῦ μαγίστρου. Ed. Studemund, Ind. lect. Vratisl. 1888/89 p. 12–14).

Berlin, Königl. Bibl., Phillipps. 1530; s. XVI.
= Ms. Phill. 1530 (*Census*: 30, nr [0126]).

Dioscurides:
(f. 1) *De materia medica* (alphab. Expl. ὑπὸ σκορπίου ἄπονοι διαμένουσιν = Spr. 284, 2).
(f. 219^{v}) *De venenis eorumque praecautione et medicatione.*
(f. 230) *De iis, quae virus eiaculantur, animalibus libellus, in quo et de rabioso cane.*

Berlin, Königl. Bibl., Phillipps. 1531 (Meerm. 223); s. XVI.
= Ms. Phill. 1531 (*Census*: 30, nr [0127]).
See also **Venedig, Bibl. Josephi de Aromatariis** below (p. 167) about Aretaeus and (p. 168) about Theophilus.

Aretaeus:
(f. 1) *De causis et signis acutorum morborum libri II* (Inc. περὶ τετάνου. σπασμοὶ οἱ τέτανοι).

(f. 16[v]) *De causis et signis diuturnorum morborum libri II.*
(f. 48[v]) *De curatione acutorum morborum libri II.*
(f. 81[v]) *De curatione diuturnorum morborum libri II* (Expl. σχεδὸν τὰ = K. 322, 4).
Theophilus: (f. 91) *De urinis.*
Ioannes Zacharias Actuarius: (f. 98[v]) *De urinis libri VII.*
Mercurius monachus: (f. 230) *De pulsibus* (»Mercurius?« Inc. Ἄψαι τοῦ σφυγμοῦ μετὰ τῶν τεσσάρων δακτύλων. Expl. καὶ τὰ τούτοις περιεχόμενα. *Vgl.* Daremberg, Not. et Extr. I p. 143 sq.).

Berlin, Königl. Bibl., Phillipps. 1532 (ol. Meerman. 225); s. XVI.
= Ms. Phill. 1532 (*Census*: 30, nr [0128]).

Philagrius: *Excerpta* (In Anonymi opere περὶ οὔρων commemorantur Σχόλια περὶ οὔρων Philagrii).
Aretaeus:
De causis et signis diuturnorum morborum libri II.
De curatione acutorum morborum libri II.
De curatione diuturnorum morborum libri II (Expl. *wie* [Berol. Phill.] 1531).
Oribasius: (f. 1[v]) *Medicae collectiones ad Iulianum* (L. XXIV. XXV).
Aretaeus: (f. 77) *De causis et signis acutorum morborum libri II.*
Anon. comm.: (f. 154) Hippokrates, *Aphorismi* (Anon. comm. in Hipp. Aph.).
Stephanus Atheniensis: (f. 173) *De febrium differentiis ex ore Theophili* (Inc. Ἡ μὲν παράδοσις ἡ περὶ τῶν πυρετῶν σύντομός ἐστι. Expl. οἷα τῶν ταριχευομένων σωμάτων. »Congruunt fere cum Palladii comm. de febribus«).
Severus: (f. 177) *De instrumentis infusoriis seu clysteribus ad Timotheum* (*Vgl.* Daremberg Not. et Extr. I p. 148).
Theophilus: (f. 180[v]) *De alvi excrementis.*

Berlin, Königl. Bibl., Phillipps. 1533; s. XVII.
= Ms. Phill. 1533 (*Census*: 30, nr [0129]).
See also **1533 (ol. Meerm. 226)** below.

Apollonius Citiensis:
(f. 90) *Commentarius in Hippocratis de articulis, libri III* (Liber I).
(f. 121) *Commentarius in Hippocratis de articulis, libri III* (Liber II).
(f. 135) *Commentarius in Hippocratis de articulis, libri III* (Liber III).

Berlin, Königl. Bibl., Phillipps. 1533 (ol. Meerm. 226); s. XVI, XVII.
Same as **1533** above.
= Ms. Phill. 1533.

Oribasius: (f. 1) *Medicae collectiones ad Iulianum* (L. XLVI–XLVIII fine mutil.).
Soranus: (f. 115) *De signis fracturarum.*

Berlin, Königl. Bibl., Phillipps. 1534 (Meerm. 229); s. XVI ex.
= Ms. Phill. 1534 (*Census*: 30, nr [0130]).

Aëtius Amidenus: *Iatricorum libri XVI.*

Berlin, Königl. Bibl., Phillipps. 1535 (ol. Meerm. 229); s. XV ex.
= Ms. Phill. 1535 (*Census*: 30, nr [0131]).

Alexander Trallianus: *Therapeutica. Libri XII.*

Berlin, Königl. Bibl., Phillipps. 1536 (ol. Meerm. 231); s. XVI.
= Ms. Phill. 1536 (*Census*: 30, nr [0132]).
See also **Montpellier, Bibliothèque de l'école** (*Vgl.* **Montfaucon, II p. 1199)** below (p. 83).

Rufus:
(f. 1), *De medicamentis purgantibus.*
(f. 9v) *De vesicae renumque affectibus.*
(f. 22)*De corporis humani appellationibus.*
(f. 30v med.) *Nomenclatura rerum ad hominem pertinentium. Libri III.*

Berlin, Königl. Bibl., Phillipps. 1538 (ol. Meerm. 233); s. XV ex.
= Ms. Phill. 1538 (*Census*: 30, nr [0134]).

Cleopatra: (f. 390v) *De mensuris et ponderibus* (Ἐκ τῶν Κλεοπ. Κοσμιτικῶν π. στ. κ. μέτρ.).

Berlin, Königl. Bibl., Phillipps. 1539; s. XVI.
= Ms. Phill. 1539 (*Census*: 30, nr [0135]).

Diodorus: (f. 3v) *De mensuris et ponderibus.*

Berlin, Königl. Bibl., Phillipps. 1540; s. XVI.
= Ms. Phill. 1540 (*Census*: 31, nr [0136]).
See also **Phillipps. 1540 (ol. Meerm. 236)** below.

Stephanus Ἀρχιατρὸς τῶν Μαγγάνων, Zosimus Panopolita: (f. 5) *Excerpta* (Περὶ ἀσβέστου. Inc. λαβὲ ἐκ τῶν τεσσάρων στοιχείων ἀρσενικοῦ.
Cleopatra: (f. 11^v med.) *De mensuris et ponderibus.*
Synesius: (f. 24) *Ad Dioscorum, scholia in librum Democriti*).
Stephanus Alexandrinus: (f. 29) *De sacra divinaque arte auri faciendi.*
Zosimus Panopolita: (f. 63) *Gemini commentarii de aqua divina.*

Berlin, Königl. Bibl., Phillipps. 1540 (ol. Meerm. 236); s. XVI.
Same as **1540** above.
= Ms. Phill. 1540.

Zosimus Panopolita: (f. 69) *Liber de virtute et compositione aquarum.*

Berlin, Königl. Bibl., Phillipps. 1547; s. XVI.
= Ms. Phill. 1547 (*Census*: 31, nr [0137]).

Soranus: (f. 120) *De ponderibus et mensuris* (Inc. Τῶν τοίνυν μέτρων καὶ σταθμῶν).

Berlin, Königl. Bibl., Phillipps. 1557; s. XVI.
= Ms. Phill. 1557 (*Census*: 31, nr [0138]).

Nemesius Emesenus: (f. 1) *De natura hominis* (Inc. mutil. [τοί]νυν ὡς ἐν εἰκόνι = Migne Patrol. 40 p. 529, 16).

Berlin, Königl. Bibl., Phillipps. 1558; s. XVI.
= Ms. Phill. 1558 (*Census*: 31, nr [0139]).

Alexander Aphrodisiensis: (f. 25) *Problematum physicorum et medicorum eclogae. Libri V* (Excerpta ex Alex. Aphr. naturalibus et moralibus ed. L. Spengel Monachii 1842).

Berlin, Königl. Bibl., Phillipps. 1562; s. XVI.
= Ms. Phill. 1562 (*Census*: 31, nr [0140]).

Constantinus Meliteniota: (f. 80) *De antidotis libri II* (Inscr. Αὗται αἱ ἀντίδοτοι ἐμετεγκομίσθησαν ἐκ τῶν Περσῶν εἰς τὴν Ἑλλάδα. Inc. Ἀντίδοτος διαφορητικὸν πνευμάτων παντὸς τοῦ σώματος. Remedia νγ').

Berlin, Königl. Bibl., Phillipps. 1566 (ol. Meerm. 269); s. XVI.
= Ms. Phill. 1566 (*Census*: 31, nr [0141]).

Theophilus: (f. 23v) *De alvi excrementis.*

Berlin, Königl. Bibl., Phillipps. 1568 (ol. Meerm. 271); s. XVI.
= Ms. Phill. 1568 (*Census*: 31, nr [0143]).

Oribasius: (f. 1) *Ad Eunapium de parabilibus medicamentis. Libri IV* (L. I 14–17).
Herophilus Sophista: (f. 22) *De alimentis, quae singulis mensibus sumenda aut vitanda sunt* (»Valde differt ab Ideleri editione«).

Berlin, Königl. Bibl., Phillipps. 1570; s. XVI.
= Ms. Phill. 1570 (*Census*: 31, nr [0144]).

Neophytus Prodromenus: (f. 55) *Remediorum collectio alphabetica.*
Paulus Aegineta: (f. 70) *De succedaneis, ex Galeno.*

Berlin, Königl. Bibl., Phillipps. 1571; s. XVI.
= Ms. Phill. 1571 (*Census*: 32, nr [0145]).
See also **1571 (ol. Meerm. 279)** below.

Athenaeus: (f. 9) *Synopsis de urinis* (Sine auctoris nomine).

Berlin, Königl. Bibl., Phillipps. 1571 (ol. Meerm. 279); s. XVI.
Same as **1571** above.
= Ms. Phill. 1571.

Paulus Aegineta: (f. 4v) *Excerpta varia* (Π. φλεβοτομίας. Inc. Φλεβοτομία λέγεται φλεβὸς ὀρθῶν τμῆμα. Expl. μακρονοσίαν σημαίνει, οὐ θάνατον).
Theodoretus: (f. 13v) *Antidota* (Ἡ λεγομένη ἀνακάρδιος).

Berlin, Königl. Bibl., Phillipps. 1576 (Meerm. 286); s. XVI.
= Ms. Phill. 1576 (*Census*: 32, nr [0146]).

Melampus: (f. 23v) *De naevis corporis.*

Berlin, Königl. Bibl., Phillipps. 1577 (Meerm. 287); s. XV.
= Ms. Phill. 1577 (*Census*: 32, nr [0147]).

Harpocration: (f. 186–198) *De facultatibus naturalibus animalium et herbarum et lapidum.*
Hermes Trismegistus: (f. 186–198) *Kyranides.*

Berlin, Königl. Bibl., Phillipps. 1581 (ol. Meerm. 297); s. XVI.
= Ms. Phill. 1581 (*Census*: 32, nr [0148]).

Oribasius: (f. 289ᵛ) *Conspectus ad Eustathium filium. Libri II* (Π. ὑδάτων = Dbg.-Buss. V p. 192–193, 6).

Berlin, Königl. Bibl., Phillipps. 1582; s. XV.
= Ms. Phill. 1582 (*Census*: 32, nr [0149]).

Ioannes Zacharias Actuarius:
(f. 1) *De urinis libri VII.*
(f. 111) *De spiritu animali libri II.*
(f. 159) *De methodo medendi Libri VI.*

Berlin, Königl. Bibl., Phillipps. 1583; s. XV.
= Ms. Phill. 1583 (*Census*: 32, nr [0150]).
See also **1583 (ol. Meerm. 300)** below.

Lucas: (f. 31) *Excerpta varia*.
Paulus Aegineta: (f. 65ᵛ) *De succedaneis, ex Galeno.*
Aëtius Amidenus: (f. 101) *Excerpta varia* (Π. οὔρων, π. σφυγμῶν).
Taronitus (?): (f. 104) *Excerpta* (Ἀντίδοτος λίθων θρυπτικὴ καὶ διουρητικὴ συντεθεῖσα παρὰ κυροῦ Κωνσταντίνου τοῦ Ταρωνείτου).
Beniaminus: (f. 105ᵛ) *Excerpta* (Φάρμακα).

Berlin, Königl. Bibl., Phillipps. 1583 (ol. Meerm. 300); s. XV.
Same as **1583** above.
= Ms. Phill. 1583.

Nicolaus Myrepsus: (f. 1) *De compositione medicamentorum, alphabetice* (Sine auctoris nomine). »Phillipps. 1583 hat mit diesem Werke nichts zu tun ...« Treu.

Bern, Stadtbibliothek
Now Burgerbibliothek Bern/Bibliothèque de la Bourgeoisie de Berne

Bern, Stadtbibliothek, 459; s. XV.

Rufus:
(f. 1) *De corporis humani appellationibus.*
(f. 23) *Nomenclatura rerum ad hominem pertinentium. Libri III.*

Bologna, Bibl. Comunale
Now Biblioteca Comunale dell'Archiginnasio

Bologna, Bibl. Comunale, Bonon. A I 13; s. XVI.
= Biblioteca Comunale dell'Archiginnasio, A 13 (*Census*: 34, nr [0157]).

Nemesius Emesenus: (f. 1) *De natura hominis.*

Bologna, Bibl. Universitaria

Bologna, Bibl. Universitaria, Bonon. 457 vol. XXIV nr 1; s. XVII.

Cleopatra: (f. 2) *De mensuris et ponderibus* (Inc. Ἡ μνᾶ ὄνομα ἔχει).

Bologna, Bibl. Universitaria, Bonon. 1808; s. XV.

Aëtius Amidenus: (f. 6) *Iatricorum libri XVI* (L. II 15–20. 22. 24–26. 30–39. 196 usque ad p. 41, 17 Ald. et L. I p. 7, 17–10, 17).
Oribasius: (f. 30^v) *Excerpta varia* (φουλ^{ιγ} σκευασία).
Theopompus: (f. 32^v) *Excerpta* (Θυμίαμα μοσχάτον).
Pamphilus: (f. 33) *Excerpta* (Θυμίαμα ῥοδάτον τοῦ ἐπισκόπου Π.).
Aëtius Amidenus: (f. 35^v) *Iatricorum libri XVI* (Frgm. L. III 114. 115. 116. 93).
Gregorius Theologus: (f. 42) *Alatium.*
Lucas: (f. 42) *Compositio salsi intinctus.*
Aëtius Amidenus:
(f. 43^v) *Iatricorum libri XVI* (L. III 19 p. 50^v usque ad διαίρεσις; subicitur καὶ ἔρινον μαλακὸν βεβρεγμένον – οὕτως σαρκοῖ ἄριστα).
(f. 44^v) *Iatricorum libri XVI* (Ex l. III 22 et l. I litt. Δ et E).
(f. 80) *Iatricorum libri XVI* (L. III 57–64. 66–69. 70. 71. 74–79. L. V 133–137. 140).
Philagrius: (f. 102) *Excerpta* (Διαφορητικὸν βρογκοκήλων καὶ σκληριῶν, θαυμάσιον φάρμακον).
Esdras Propheta: (f. 124^v) *Antidotus Esdrae.*
Asclepiades: (f. 128) *Excerpta varia* (Inc. Ὁ δὲ Ἀσκληπιάδης σκευάζεσθαι κελεύει τὴν πικρὰν ὡς Θεμίσων).
Aëtius Amidenus:
(f. 159) *Iatricorum libri XVI* (L. I p. 3–7, 49; subiciuntur f. 169^v ταύτην ἱερὰν καλοῦσι – παρβάτως).
(f. 170^v) *Iatricorum libri XVI* (Ex l. III 110–113. 138. 139. 141. 143).
Dioscurides: (f. 174) *Excerpta* (Κοινά βοηθήματα τῶν νηπὰ [sic] περίοδον παροξυνομένων).

Aëtius Amidenus: *Iatricorum libri XVI*:
(f. 175) Frgm.
(f. 182ᵛ) Ex. l. VI 24. VI 23. 28.
(f. 201) Ex l. IV 3–20. VII 98–101.
(f. 225) L. IV 21–26. VI 66–79. 80. 81. 83–86. 88. 93–95. VIII 12. 13– 15. 9. 16. 17. 19. 20. 22–24.
(f. 253ᵛ) Ex l. VIII 40–42.
(f. 262ᵛ) Ex l. VI 50–53.
Rufus: (f. 267) *Excerpta varia* (Χρῖσμα ἐπεργὸν ἐντεῖνον τὸ αἰδοῖον).
Oribasius: (f. 267) *Excerpta varia* (Πρὸς πάρεσιν τοῦ αἰδοίου μάλιστα γερόντων).
Philagrius: (f. 267ᵛ) *Excerpta* (Περὶ ὀνειράξεων [l. ὀνειρώξεων]. »Ex Aetio?« Wellmann).

Bologna, Bibl. Universitaria, Bonon. 2294; s. XV.

Alexander Aphrodisiensis: (f. 61) *Quarundam difficultatum solutiones* (Quaestionum libri IV).

Bologna, Bibl. Universitaria, Bonon. 2911; s. XVI.

S. Basilius: (f. 73) *De hominis generatione. Libri III.*

Bologna, Bibl. Universitaria, Bonon. 3632; s. XV.

Paulus Aegineta: (f. 16ᵛ) *Excerpta varia* (Imaginum quae P. Aeg. chirurgiam illustrant index).
Archelaus: (f. 43) *Fragmentum.*
Magnus Emesenus, **Theophilus**:
(f. 51ᵛ) *De urinis.*
(f. 57) *De urinis* (Inc. Τῶν οὔρων αἱ διαφοραὶ πολλαί. Expl. κατὰ τὰ εἰρημένα. »Concordat cum commentatione de urinis, quam Ideler Anonymo tribuit, ab initio usque ad II p. 315, 20«).
Aëtius Amidenus: *Iatricorum libri*:
(f. 59) Ex l. V 28–44 p. 80–81 Ald.
(f. 62ᵛ) Ex l. V 45.
Marcellinus: (f. 65) *De pulsibus* (Inc. Σφυγμὸν θήγειν καὶ περὶ σφυγμῶν ὅσα χρὴ μαθήν = Zeile 2 Schoene. Expl. τὴν ἐπιπλοκὴν ἔχων = Zeile 485 Sch.).
Aëtius Amidenus: *Iatricorum libri*:
(f. 67ᵛ) L. V 26.
(f. 71) Frgm. ex l. I.
(f. 92) L. II 13–36.
(f. 97ᵛ) L. II 4–82 p. 16ᵛ–31.

Paulus Aegineta: (f. 114ᵛ) *Excerpta varia* (Capita nonnulla P. Aeg. tributa).
Aëtius Amidenus: *Iatricorum libri*:
(f. 114ᵛ) Capita Aëtio tributa.
(f. 125) L. II 198–204. 208. 209–214 p. 41–42.
(f. 127) L. II 220. 228. 230. 235. 236. 239. 241–245. 254–257. 260. 263. 269. L. III 138–140. 142. II 223. 226. III 143. 148. 149. 150. 158. III 160–163. 166. 170.
(f. 132) De febrium differentiis.
Palladius: (f. 132) *Stephani philosophi vel Palladii synopsis de febribus* (Initium tantum [Ideler p. 107, 1–17] comparari potest cum libro Palladii).
Taronitus (?): (f. 138) *Excerpta* (Ἐπίθεμα καταρκοικον [sic !]).
Aëtius Amidenus: *Iatricorum libri*:
(f. 143) Π. συνουσίας ἀμέτρου καὶ ἐμμέτρου. Inc. Φυσικῶν ἔργων.
(f. 172–181) Περὶ γυναικῶν παθῶν μητρικῶν καὶ τῶν ὁμοίων.
Damascius: (f. 189ᵛ) *Excerpta* (Περὶ τῶν ἀντιδότων. Στήλη τῆς ἱερᾶς Δαμασκηνοῦ).
Taronitus (?): (f. 189ᵛ) *Excerpta* (Ἀντίδοτος).
Oribasius: (f. 204) *Excerpta varia* (Περὶ τῶν ἀντιδότων cap. ρλθ', extremum ἀληθυριακὸν Ὀρ.).
Iustus: (f. 206) *Excerpta* (Περὶ τῶν ἱερῶν καὶ πικρῶν ἀντιδότων, cap. ιθ' extr.: Ἱερὰ Ἰούστου κ^{θ}'. *Wohl aus* Aët. III 116).
Alexander Trallianus: (f. 207) *Excerpta* (Ἱερὰ ἀντίδοτος).
Paulus Aegineta: (f. 209ᵛ) *Excerpta varia* (Ἀρχὴ π. τροχῆσκον [*l.* τροχίσκων] capp. 77; cap. 2–41 concordant cum lib. VII 12 P. Aeg.).
Photius monachus: (f. 217) *Excerpta* (Ζουλάπιον).
Gregorius Theologus: (f. 228) *Alatium*.
Theosebius: (f. 232ᵛ) *Excerpta* (Ὑποθέματα δυσεντερικὰ καὶ ἐπιθέματα).
Aëtius Amidenus: (f. 233ᵛ) *Excerpta varia*.
Asclepiades: (f. 233ᵛ) *Excerpta varia* (Καθαρτικῶν συγγραφή).
Aëtius Amidenus: (f. 236) *Iatricorum libri XVI* (L. IV 101–104. 108).
Paulus Aegineta: (f. 259) *Excerpta varia* (Χρήσματος ἀπὸ τοῦ κόδητος [sic !] τοῦ Π.).
Theophilus: (f. 262) *Excerpta* (Inscr. Περὶ θεραπείας ψυχῆς; *vgl. f.* 16. Inc. Ἔλεγον οἱ πατέρες, ὅτι μόναχός τις ἐρχόμενός ἐστι. Expl. προσκύνει [?] τὸν δεσπότην Χριστόν).
Rufus: (f. 265) *Excerpta varia* (Περὶ αἵματος).
Ptolemaeus: *Excerpta*:
(f. 317ᵛ) Ἐκ τῆς γενεθλιακῆς βίβλου τῆς ἀποτελεσματικῆς μερικὰ περί τε ἀρρένων καὶ θηλέων τέκνων.
(f. 320ᵛ) Περὶ τῶν ιβ' ζωδίων.

Dioscurides: (f. 377–378) *De materia medica* (Imagines plantarum, quae ut in ind. f. 16^{v} adnotatum est ad D. referenda sunt: Δ. τὰ βότανα ἱστορημένα. Apographon cod. Vindob. med. 1 [below p. 178]).

Paulus Aegineta: (f. 379) *Excerpta varia* (Ad titulum περὶ δεσμῶν imagines).

Ioannes Zacharias Actuarius: (f. 380) *De animalibus nocentibus* (Ὀκταρίου).

Paulus Aegineta: (f. 382. 383^{v}) *Excerpta varia* (Ad titulum περὶ δεσμῶν imagines).

Dioscurides:

(f. 385–416^{v}) *De materia medica* (Imagines plantarum sim. f. 377–378).

(f. 385–416^{v}) *Excerpta*.

(f. 417^{v}) *De materia medica* (Imagines plantarum sim. f. 377–378).

Apollonius Citiensis: (f. 419–434) *Commentarius in Hippocratis de articulis, libri III* (Imagines).

Paulus Aegineta: (f. 419–434^{v}) *Excerpta varia* (Ad tit. de repositionibus, lib. VI c. 114. 102. 118. 117 imagines; *vgl. Apollon. Citiensis*).

Hermes Trismegistus:

(f. 435^{v}) *Ad Asclepium de plantis XII zodiaci signorum.*

Ad Asclepium de plantis VII planetarum.

Bologna, Bibl. Universitaria, Bonon. 3633; s. XV.

Diocles: (f. 126) *Hippocratis vel, ut alii volunt, Dioclis epistula ad Ptolemaeum Aegypti regem.*

Bologna, Bibl. Universitaria, Bonon. 3635; s. XIV.

Alexander Aphrodisiensis:

(f. 1) *Problematum physicorum et medicorum eclogae. Libri V* (Libri I et II).

(f. 51^{v})*Problematum physicorum et medicorum eclogae. Libri V* (Excerpta. Inc. Οἱ μὲν πλεῖστοι τῶν παλαιοτέρων ἰατρῶν. Expl. ἐξευρεῖν τὴν γονὴν).

Cassius iatrosophistes: (f. 79) *Quaestiones medicae et problemata physica.*

Bologna, Bibl. Universitaria, Bonon. 3636; s. XIV–XV.

Paulus Aegineta: (f. 61^{v}) *Excerpta varia* (Κατὰ στοιχεῖον ἁπλαῖ θεραπεῖαι. Inc. Ἄβροτα διατηρεῖ σκωλύκων. Expl. καὶ γάλακτι γυναικείῳ ἐγγλυόμενον).

Diocles: (f. 127) *Ad Antigonum regem epistula de tuenda valetitudine* (Sub nomine Pauli Aegin.).

Theophilus: (f. 133^{v}) *De alvi excrementis* (Expl. ἀπολείπεται τὸ διαχώρημα = Idel. I 399, 31).

Severus: (f. 134^{v}) *De instrumentis infusoriis seu clysteribus ad Timotheum.*

Paulus Aegineta: (f. 140^{v}) *Epitomae medicae libri septem* (L. III 26. 25. 52. 54. 81. L. VI 85. 86. 87. L. III 58. L. I 43–46. 51. 203. L. III 27. L. II 12).

Breslau

Breslau, Vratisl. Rhedig. bibl. urb., 34; s. XV.
Now Wrocław, Biblioteka Uniwersytecka we Wrocławiu, Rehd 34 (*Census*: 36, nr [0171]).

Nemesius Emesenus: (f. 1–54^{v}) *De natura hominis.*

Brüssel, Königl. Bibl.
Now Bruxelles, Bibliothèque royale de Belgique

Brüssel, Königl. Bibl., Bruxell. 5362–64; s. XVI.

Meletius monachus: (f. 105) *De natura hominis* (Expl. ἐν καρδίας διὰ τῆς ἀορτῆς ἀρ...).

Brüssel, Königl. Bibl., Bruxell. 11337–41; s. –.

Ioannes Zacharias Actuarius:
(f. 1) *De spiritu animali libri II.*
(f. 138^{v}. 239) *De methodo medendi Libri VI.*

Brüssel, Königl. Bibl., Bruxell. 11345–48; s. XVI.

Erotianus: (f. 1) *Vocum Hippocraticarum conlectio.*

Brüssel, Königl. Bibl., Bruxell. 11351–52; s. XVI.

Nemesius Emesenus: *De natura hominis* (Inc. cap. 2 διαφωνεῖται σχεδόν).

Brüssel, Königl. Bibl., Bruxell. 11354; s. –.

Gregorius Nyssenus: (f. 1) *De hominis opificio* (De homine capp. 30. Inc. Θεωρία τις ἡ ἀκριβωτέρα [sic]. Expl. κεκριμένην μὲν ζῶσαν).

Budapest

Budapest, Mus. nat. Hungar., 9 fol.; s. XVI.
Now Budapest, Országos Széchényi Könyvtár, Kéziratar, Fol. Graec. 9 (*Census*: 38, nr [0178]).

Oribasius:
(f. 1–10ᵛ) *Conspectus ad Eustathium filium. Libri II* (Frgm.).
(f. 11–33) *Ad Eunapium de parabilibus medicamentis. Libri IV* (Expl. τοσοῦτον ἐμβάλῃς ὄξους ὅσον μέλιτος).
(f. 23ᵛ–35ᵛ) *Medicae collectiones ad Iulianum* (L. III *z. T. in veränderter Fassung*).
(f. 35ᵛ. 36) *Excerpta varia* (Inc. Συκάμινα βάτινα. Expl. ἐπεμβάλλειν αὐτῷ).
(f. 36–65ᵛ) *Excerpta varia* (Περὶ τῆς δυνάμεως τῶν ἁπλῶν κατὰ στοιχεῖον. Inc. Ὅσα μὲν εἰδέναι τέ σε καὶ ποιεῖν. Expl. καὶ ἀδήκτως ξηραίνει).
(f. 66–158ᵛ) *Ad Eunapium de parabilibus medicamentis. Libri IV* (Expl. τοσοῦτον ἐμβάλῃς ὄξους ὅσον μέλιτος).

Cairo

Cairo, Patriarch. Alexandrin., 46 (*bei* Coxe, Mss. gr. of the Levant); s. XV.
= Αλεξάνδρεια (الإسكندرية), Πατριαρχείο, Πατριαρχική Βιβλιοθήκη Αλεξανδρείας, 36 (?) (*Census*: 39, nr [0181]).

Theophilus: *De alvi excrementis.*

Cambridge, Caius Coll.
Now Cambridge, Gonville and Caius College

Cambridge, Caius Coll., 50; s. XV/XVI.
Now 50/27 (*Census*: 40, nr [0184]).

Soranus: (f. 1) *Hippocratis genus et vita secundum Soranum.*

Cambridge, Caius Coll., 76; s. XV/XVI.
Now 76/43 (*Census*: 40, nr [0185]).

Ioannes Zacharias Actuarius: (f. 35) *De urinis libri VII.*

Cambridge, Caius Coll., 77; s. XV–XVI.
Now 77/44 (*Census*: 40, nr [0186]).

Alexander Trallianus: (f. 1) *Therapeutica. Libri XII* (*Coll. im Leydens. Periz 4° 2/9 fasc. 2*).

Cambridge, Cantabrig. Bibl. Univ.
Now Cambridge, University Library

Cambridge, Cantabrig. Bibl. Univ., 2049 (Kk V 7); s. XV–XVI.
Now Cambridge University Library Kk. 5. 7 (*Census*: 44–45, nr [0197]).

Erotianus: *Vocum Hippocraticarum conlectio.*

Cambridge, Cantabrig. Bibl. Univ., F. F. 3. 30; s. XVI.
Now Cambridge University Library Ff. 3. 30.

Alexander Aphrodisiensis: (nr 6) *Problematum physicorum et medicorum eclogae. Libri V.*
Diocles: (nr 7) *Ad Antigonum regem epistula de tuenda valetitudine.*

Cambridge, Cantabrig. Bibl. Univ., Gg I 2; s. XV.
Now Cambridge University Library Gg. 1. 2.

Epiphanius: (f. 261) *De mensuris et ponderibus* (Frgm. Expl. κουστωδία ἄνδρες ϡ).

Cambridge, Cantabrig. Bibl. Univ., L l IV 12; s. XV.
Now Cambridge University Library Ll. 4. 12.

Gregorius Nyssenus: (f. 47) *De hominis opificio.*

Cambridge, Coll. St. Johann.
Now Cambridge, St John's College

Cambridge, Coll. St. Johann., A 6; s. XV–XVI.
= St John's College, MS A. 6 (*Census*: 46, nr [0204]).

Oribasius: *Medicae collectiones ad Iulianum* (L. I–XV).

Cambridge, Trinity Coll.
Now Cambridge, Trinity College

Cambridge, Trinity Coll., 1386; s. XV. XVI.
Now Cambridge, Trinity College, O.8.11 (*Census*: 48, nr [0207]).

Ioannes Zacharias Actuarius: (f. 9) *De urinis libri VII.*

Carpentras

Carpentras, Bibl. Inguimbertine, nr. 1774; s. XVII.
See also **1774 (P. V.)** below.

Oribasius: (f. 140ᵛ) *Excerpta varia* (De ponderibus et mensuris manifestum experimentum medicum).

Carpentras, Bibl. Inguimbertine, nr. 1774 (P., V/ P. V.); s. XVII.
Same as **nr. 1774** above (*Census*: 49, nr [0209]).

Cleopatra: (f. 139) *De mensuris et ponderibus.*
Epiphanius: (f. 144) *De mensuris et ponderibus* (Frgm.).
Eusebius: (f. 162ᵛ) *De mensuris et ponderibus.*(f. 269).
Eusebius: *De mensuris et ponderibus.*
Adamantius: (f. 165) *Excerpta* (De ponderibus et mensuris).
Marcellus Sidetes: (f. 168) *De mensuris et ponderibus* (*Vgl.* f. 315).

Cheltenham

Cheltenham, Phillipps., 3084; s. XV.
Now New Haven, Yale University, Harvey Cushing/John Hay Whitney Library, Manuscript 31 vault (*Census*: 50, nr [0213]).

Dioscurides: (f. 1) *De materia medica* (Inscr. ⟨περὶ βοτανῶν⟩ καὶ ῥιζῶν καὶ χυλισμάτων καὶ σπερμάτων συνφύλλων ⟨τε καὶ⟩ φαρμάκων, κατὰ στοιχεῖον. Inc. ἀβρότονον τὸ μέγα. Expl. περὶ ὠκίμου ... πληγέντες ὑπὸ σκορπίου, ἄσωστοι διατίθενται; *vgl. den* Berolinens. Phill. [1530] [p. 17]).

Cheltenham, Phillipps., 3892 (ol. Meerm. 275); s. XV.
Now New Haven, Yale University, Harvey Cushing/John Hay Whitney Library, Manuscript 33 vault (*Census*: 50–51, nr [0214]).

Meletius monachus: (nr 1) *De natura hominis*.

Cheltenham, Phillipps., 6763; s. XV (XIV Cat. und Schenkl).
Now New Haven, Yale University, Harvey Cushing/John Hay Whitney Library, Manuscript 34 vault (*Census*: 51, nr [0217]).

Stephanus Alexandrinus: (f. 1) *In Magni sophistae librum de urinis* (Μάγνου σοφ. ἐξήγησις εἰς τὸ περὶ οὔρων καὶ ἄλλων πολλῶν παλαιῶν σοφῶν τε καὶ διδασκάλων, συντεθεῖσα παρὰ τοῦ φιλοσόφου Στεφ. τοῦ Ἀλεξ.).
Olymnius Alexandrinus:
(f. 29) *Excerpta* (Inc. Τῶν κρισίμων ἡμερῶν αἱ μὲν κατὰ σύλληψίν εἰσιν. Expl. καὶ ἐν ἐνιαυτῷ καὶ ἐν ἑπτὰ ἔτεσι).
(f. 29^{v}) *De decubitu*.

Cheltenham, Phillipps., 21975; s. IX.
Now New York, Pierpont Morgan Library, MS M 652 (*Census*: 52, nr [0219], 166).

Dioscurides:
(f. 1, 200–220, 221, 243, 270) *De materia medica* (Inc. mutil. καὶ κοιλίαν καὶ ἔμμηνα κινεῖ. alphab.).
(f. 306) *De venenis eorumque praecautione et medicatione* (Inscr. *wie im* Athous [Βιβλ. Μον. Λαύρας, Ω 75] [see p. 11]).
(f. 319^{v}) *De iis, quae virus eiaculantur, animalibus libellus, in quo et de rabioso cane*.
(f. 332^{v}) *Excerpta* (Περὶ ἀντιφαρμάκων).
Eutecnius:
(f. 360^{v}) *Paraphrasis in Nicandri Theriaca* (*vgl.* f. 338ss).
(f. 375) *Paraphrasis in Nicandri Alexipharmaca*.

Cheltenham, Phillipps., 23007; s. XV.
Now divided in three manuscripts (see *Census*: 52, nr [0220]).
Paris, Chicago, and New York, Les Enluminures, TM 540.
Provo, Brigham Young University, Lee Library, L. Tom Perry Special Collections, vault 091 G13 1475.
Paris, private collection.

Hermes Trismegistus: *Iatromathematica ad Ammonium Aegyptium* (Inc. Τὸν ἄνθρωπον, ὦ Ἄμμων, φερέκοσμον. Expl. mutil. ἐὰν δὲ σελήνης οὔσης ἐν ταύρῳ κατακλιθῇ τις Κρόνου συνόντος αὐτῇ ἢ ἀναμετροῦντος = Ideler I p. 395, 20).

Dresden, Königl. Bibl.
Now Sächsische Landesbibliothek – Staats- und Universitätsbibliothek Dresden

Dresden, Königl. Bibl., Da 5, a. 1519.
Now Москва (Moskva), Российский Государственный Архив Древних Актов (РГАДА) (Rossiiskii Gosudarstvennyi Arkhiv Drevnikh Aktov [RGADA], Russian State Archive of Ancient Documents [RGADA]), Фонд (Fond.) 1607, Dresden Da 05 (*Census*: 58, nr [0224]).

Ioannes Zacharias Actuarius:
(f. 2) *De spiritu animali libri II.*
(f. 176^{v} [vor]) *De methodo medendi libri VI.*
Paulus Aegineta: (f. 176^{v}) *De succedaneis, ex Galeno* (Frgm.).
Ioannes Zacharias Actuarius:
(f. 176^{v}) *Excerpta varia* (Περὶ σταθμῶν καὶ χαρακτήριων αὐτῶν καὶ τῶν μέτρων. »zu streichen; ist nicht von Zacharias, denn vor περὶ σταθμῶν usw. steht nicht τοῦ αὐτοῦ.« Treu).
(f. 182) *De urinis libri VII.*
Mercurius monachus: (f. 247) *De pulsibus* (Sine auctoris nomine. Inc. *wie im* [Berol.] Phillipps. [1531]) (see p. 17).
Oribasius: (f. 249) *Excerpta varia* (Περὶ οὔρων).

Dresden, Königl. Bibl., Da 57; s. XII.

Nemesius Emesenus: (f. 1) *De natura hominis.*

Dresden, Königl. Bibl., Da 58; s. XV.

Nemesius Emesenus: (f. 1) *De natura hominis* (Frgm. capp. 35–38).

Edschmiadzin

Edschmiadzin (Provinz Ararat), nr. ?; s. VIII.
= Երևան (Yerevan), Մատենադարան.Մ. Մաշտոցի անվան հին ձեռագրերի գիտահետազոտական ինստիտուտ (Matenadaran. M. Maštoc'i anvan hin jeṙagreri gitahetazotakan institut [Matenadaran. Mesrop Mashtots Institute of Ancient Manuscripts]), M 141 (*Census*: 61, nr [0233]).
See below Oxford, Bibl. Bodl., *e 19 [31.528]* (p. 93).

Dioscurides: *De materia medica* (Fragmenta libri III).

Erlangen, Universitätsbibliothek
Now Universitätsbibliothek Erlangen-Nürnberg

Erlangen, Universitätsbibliothek, Bibl. Univ., 89; s. XV.
Now Ms. A 4 (*Census*: 61, nr [0234]).

Hermes Trismegistus:
(nr 11) *De XII locorum nomenclatura et facultate.*
(nr 13) *Iatromathematica ad Ammonium Aegyptium.*
(f. 159) *De XII locorum nomenclatura et facultate.*
(f. 175^{v}) *Ad Asclepium de plantis VII planetarum.*
(f. 175^{v}) *Ad Asclepium de plantis XII zodiaci signorum.*
(f. 177^{v}) *Iatromathematica ad Ammonium Aegyptium* (Inc. Ἐν τῇ καταβολῇ τοῦ ἀνθρωπίνου σπέρματος).

Erlangen, Universitätsbibliothek, 90 (vel Erlangens. 90); s. XVI.
Now Ms. A. 3 (*Census*: 61, nr [0235]).

Philotheus: *Explicatio in Hippocratis Aphorismos* (inde ab Aph. XXIV). Inc. Τὰ διακαῆ καὶ ζέουσαν. Expl. τέλος τῶν λειπομένων Θεοφίλου φιλοσ. εἰς τοῦ Ἱππ. ἀφορισμούς).
Aëtius Amidenus: (f. 1) *Excerpta varia* (Σύνοψις τῶν τρίτων βιβλίων Ὀριβασίου τοῦ πρὸς Ἰουλ. καὶ τοῦ πρὸς Εὐστάθ. ... Γαλ. καὶ Ἀρχιγ. καὶ Ῥούφου κτλ.» Cod. descriptus est ex Ald. a. 1534«).
Theophilus: (nr. 90) *Commentarius in Hippocratis aphorismos* (Inde ab aphor. XXIV).

Escurial
Now San Lorenzo de El Escorial,
Biblioteca del Real Monastero de San Lorenzo del Escorial

Escurial, Scorial. – (Puschm. I p. 90).
Verbleib unbekannt.
= **Φ. I. 2** below (p. 37) (*Census*: 62 nr [0236]).

Alexander Trallianus: *Epistula de lumbricis.*

Escurial, Scorial. III. R. 3; s. XI.
= R.III.3 (*Census*: 62, nr [0238]).

Dioscurides:
(f. 1) *De materia medica* (Exordium ducit ex fragmento cap. 20 [c. 22 editionis] libri II. – Libri VI).
(f. 129ᵛ) *De venenis eorumque praecautione et medicatione.*
Alexander Trallianus: (f. 141ᵛ) *Excerpta* (Medicamina sine auctoris nomine; *vgl.* Dioscuridis de mat. med. libri V ed. M. Wellmann, vol. II p. XII).

Escurial, Scorial. R. I. 12; s. XV.

Paulus Aegineta:
De succedaneis, ex Galeno (hinter Ἐπιτ. Lib. VI).
De mensuris et ponderibus (hinter Περὶ ἀντεμβαλλομένων).
Aëtius Amidenus: (f. 1) *Iatricorum libri XVI* (L. IX–XII).
Paulus Aegineta: (f. 91ᵛ) *Epitomae medicae libri septem* (Liber VI).
Aëtius Amidenus: (f. 135ᵛ) *Iatricorum libri XVI* (L. XIII–XVI).

Escurial, Scorial. Σ. I. 12; s. XVI.

Hypatus: (f. 51) *Interpretatio partium corporis* (Sine auctoris nomine. Inc. Τὸ ἁπαλὸν βρέγμα. Expl. ταρσὸν καὶ πλατύπεδίον [sic]. *Vgl.* Rufus ed. Ruelle p. 599).
Rufus: (f. 51) *De corporis humani appellationibus* (Frgm. Sine inscriptione).

Escurial, Scorial. Σ. I. 17; s. XV.

Dioscurides:
(f. 1) *De materia medica* (alphab.).
(f. 188) *De venenis eorumque praecautione et medicatione* (Inscr. *wie im* Athous [Βιβλ. Μον. Λαύρας, Ω 75] [see p. 11]).
(f. 197ᵛ) *De iis, quae virus eiaculantur, animalibus libellus, in quo et de rabioso cane.*
Eutecnius:
(f. 212) *Paraphrasis in Nicandri Theriaca.*
(f. 232ᵛ) *Paraphrasis in Nicandri Alexipharmaca.*
(f. 246) *Paraphrasis in Oppiani Halieutica.*
(f. 259ᵛ) *Paraphrasis in Dionysii Ixeutica.*

Escurial, Scorial. Σ. II. 3; s. XVI.

Nicolaus Myrepsus: (f. 12) *De compositione medicamentorum, alphabetice.*

Escurial, Scorial. Σ. II. 10; s. X.

Stephanus Atheniensis: (f. 1) *In aphorismos Hippocratis commentarius* (Inc. ⟨Αἱ⟩ μεταβολαὶ τῶν ὡρέων. Expl. φύσει ἀνώμαλον εἶναι τὸ φθινόπωρον).

Escurial, Scorial. Σ. III. 17; s. XVI.

Aëtius Amidenus:
(f. 1) *Excerpta varia* (Frgm. Synopsis simpl. Gal. medicamentorum liber II).
(f. 9) *Excerpta varia* (Libri I excerpt.).
(f. 102) *Iatricorum libri XVI* (Frgm. l. I inc. αἱ διαφοραὶ τῶν κατὰ μέρος ἐνεργειῶν. Expl. στρόφους πραΰνει).
Theophilus: (f. 126ᵛ) *De arte medica.*
Nemesius Emesenus: (f. 141) *De natura hominis* (Frgm. Inc. Μέχρι τοῦ βάθους διϊκνεῖσθαι πέφυκεν ἡ ὄψις. Expl. ἐπειδὴ δὲ τῶν αἰσθητικῶν ἡδονῶν οἱ μὲν ἄλλαις ...).
Aëtius Amidenus: (f. 220) *Excerpta varia* (Libri I excerpt.).

Escurial, Scorial. T. II. 12; s. XVI.

Dioscurides: (f. 4–138) *De materia medica* (alphab.).

Escurial, Scorial T. II 14; s. XVI.
Same as **T. II. 14** below (*Census*: 63, nr [0250]).

Hermes Trismegistus: (f. 178ᵛ) *Excerpta varia* (Ἀντίδοτος ἡ καλουμένη Ἑρμοῦ ἐκ τῶν ἀδύτων τοῦ Ἑρμοῦ εἰς μεμφίην παρεχώρησεν. »Ex Isaaci Iudaei libro τῶν ἐφοδίων videtur desumpta«).

Escurial, Scorial. T. II. 14; s. XVII.
See also **T. II 14** above.

Ioannes Damascenus: *Excerpta* (Πόμα ἤτοι βοήθημα διὰ πειρας μεγάλης δόκιμον · ἄνθη τῆς βιόλας. »Ex Isaaci libro videntur desumpta. Cf. cod. Matrit. 166. f. 212.« Wellmann).
Stephanus Atheniensis: (f. 177) *De febrium differentiis ex ore Theophili* (Inc. Ὁπηνίκα γὰρ = Ideler I p. 109, 35. Expl. πρὸς τὴν διαφορὰν τῆς ὕλης).
Palladius: (f. 177) *Stephani philosophi vel Palladii synopsis de febribus* (Frgm. Inc. Ὁπηνίκα γὰρ πλεονάσει. Expl. πρὸς τὴν διαφορὰν τῆς ὕλης. *Vgl.* Ideler p. 109, 35 sq).
Ioannes Zacharias Actuarius: (f. 192) *De urinis libri VII.*
Aëtius Amidenus: (f. 199ᵛ) *Iatricorum libri XVI* (L. IV et V).

Escurial, Scorial. Υ. I. 9; s. XVI.

Alexander Aphrodisiensis: (f. 5) *Problematum physicorum et medicorum eclogae. Libri IV* (Frgm. Libri II).

Escurial, Scorial. Υ. III. 14; s. XV.

Paulus Aegineta: (f. 1v) *De succedaneis, ex Galeno.*
Ioannes Zacharias Actuarius: (f. 6v) *De methodo medendi libri VI* (Frgm.).
Theophilus: (f. 22) *De alvi excrementis.*
Theophilus: (f. 31) *De urinis.*
Magnus Emesenus: (f. 55) *De urinis.*
Paulus Aegineta: (f. 77v) *De succedaneis, ex Galeno.*
Ioannes Damascenus: (f. 89) *Excerpta* (Ex Isaaci libro).
Paulus Aegineta: (f. 188) *Epitomae medicae libri septem* (Liber VII init. mutil.).
Diocles: (f. 236) *Ad Antigonum regem epistula de mensuris et ponderibus* (Inc. Τὸ γράμμα ἄγει κεράτια ϛʹ. Expl. τοῦ ἐλαίου ℔ ιηʹ).
Heliodorus: (f. 236v) *De mensuris et ponderibus.*

Escurial, Scorial. y. I. 8; s. XVI.

Theophilus: (f. 1) *Commentarius in Hippocratis aphorismos.*
Palladius: (f. 82) *Scholia in Hippocratis de popularibus morbis librum sextum, sectiones VIII.*
Aretaeus:
(f. 162) *De causis et signis acutorum morborum libri II* (initio mutil. Inc. *wie im* [Berol.] Phillipps. 1531 l. I 8 [see p. 17]).
(f. 181v) *De causis et signis diuturnorum morborum libri II.*
(f. 218) *De curatione acutorum morborum libri II.*
(f. 252v) *De curatione diuturnorum morborum libri II* (scatet lacunis).

Escurial, Scorial. y. I. 9; s. XVI.

Oribasius: (f. 1) *Conspectus ad Eustathium filium. Libri II.*
Erotianus: (f. 158) *Vocum Hippocraticarum conlectio.*

Escurial, Scorial. y. I. 15, s. XVI.

Meletius monachus:
(f. 1) *De natura hominis* (Frgm. Τὴν ἀρχὴν δὲ ἀπὸ τῶν τοῦ θαυμασίου πρεσβυτέρου ἡμῶν. Expl. τὰ ἔργα σου, κύριε, πάντα ἐν σοφίᾳ ἐποίησας).
(f. 73v) *De anima* (»Περὶ ψυχῆς Meletii esse videtur«. Wellmann. Inc. Ὁ περὶ ψυχῆς ὅδε λόγος οὐ τὸ τί ἐστιν ἡ ψυχὴ κατ᾽ οὐσίαν διδάσκει. Expl. οἱ γνῶσιν ἐν συνέσει κατωρθωκότες).

Escurial, Scorial. y. III. 18; s. XV *und* XVI.

Stephanus Alexandrinus: (f. 86) *De mundo. Libri IX.*

Escurial, Scorial. Φ. I. 2; s. XVI.
See also above (p. 33) **Scorial. – (Puschm. I p. 90)** and below **Φ. I. 2 (?)**.

Rufus:
(f. 1) *De corporis humani appellationibus.*
(f. 8^{v}) *Nomenclatura rerum ad hominem pertinentium. Libri III.*
Oribasius: (f. 16^{v}. 43^{v}) *Medicae collectiones ad Iulianum* (L. XXIV. XXV).
Africanus: (f. 72) *De ponderibus et mensuris.*
Paulus Aegineta: (f. 73^{v}) *Epitomae medicae libri septem* (L. VI 8 ἀνωτέρω τῶν κατὰ φύσιν τριχῶν. Expl. τὸν ἁρμόζοντα δεῖ ποιεῖσθαι χειρισμόν).
Aelius Promotus: (f. 139) *Dynameron* (*Apographon des* [Venet.] Marcian. [295] [below p. 171]).
Alexander Trallianus: (f. 196 *und* 308) *Therapeutica. Libri XII* (Frgm. *Apographon des* [Venet.] Marcian. 295).

Escurial, Scorial. Φ. I. 2 (?); s. XVI.
Same as **Φ. I. 2** above.

Alexander Trallianus: (f. 191) *De oculis. Libri III* (*vgl.* Puschm. I p. 90).

Escurial, Scorial. Φ. I. 6; s. XVI.

Aëtius Amidenus: (f. 1 = 153) *Iatricorum libri XVI* (L. IX–XVI).

Escurial, Scorial. Φ. I. 10; s. XVI.

Meletius monachus: (f. 189^{v}) *De anima* (Frgm.).
Diocles: (f. 197) *Ad Antigonum regem epistula de tuenda valetitudine.*
Dioscurides: (f. 205) *Excerpta.*

Escurial, Scorial. Φ. I. 11; s. XVI.

Cleopatra: (f. 15^{v}) *De mensuris et ponderibus.*
Stephanus Alexandrinus: (f. 36^{v}) *De sacra divinaque arte auri faciendi.*

Escurial, Scorial. Φ. II. 15; s. XIV.

Aëtius Amidenus: *Iatricorum libri XVI:*
(f. 1) Frgm. l. XVI 72 π. μύλης.
(f. 7) Frgm. l. XIII 63–70.
(f. 8) L. XII 37 προσαγέσθω – XVI.

Escurial, Scorial. Φ. III. 7; s. XIV.

Dioscurides: (f. 5ᵛ) *De mensuris et ponderibus* (Frgm. Inc. Τὸ κεράμιον λίτρας οβ').
Leo: (f. 186ᵛ) *De natura hominis.*

Escurial, Scorial. Φ. III. 11; s. XIV–XV, XIV. XV, XIV *und* XV.

Theophilus: (f. 1) *De urinis.*
Gregorius Nyssenus: (f. 49ᵛ) *De pulsibus* (Περὶ σφυγμῶν καὶ ἑτέρων κινήσεως τοῦ σώματος).

Escurial, Scorial. Φ. III. 12; s. XV.

Ioannes Zacharias Actuarius:
(f. 1) *Excerpta varia* (Inc. Ξανθῆς χολῆς εἰς κένωσιν προκειμένης).
(f. 12) *De urinis libri VII.*
(f. 130) *De spiritu animali libri II.*
(f. 175) *De methodo medendi libri VI.*
(f. 346) *De animalibus nocentibus.*
(f. 352ᵛ. 396. 411. 415) *De methodo medendi libri VI.*
Paulus Aegineta:
(f. 421) *Epitomae medicae libri septem medicae libri septem* (Liber II).
(f. 467) *De succedaneis, ex Galeno.*

Escurial, Scorial. X. I. 11; s. XVI.

Nemesius Emesenus: (f. 1) *De natura hominis.*
Alexander Aphrodisiensis: (f. 64) *De nutritione et augmento.*

Escurial, Scorial. X. II. 2; s. XVI.

Epiphanius: (f. 129ᵛ) *De duodecim gemmis panno sacerdotis infibulatis.*

Escurial, Scorial. X. II. 9; a. 1564.

Nemesius Emesenus: (f. 1) *De natura hominis* (fine mutil.).

Escurial, Scorial. Ψ. I. 13; s. XVI.

Stephanus Alexandrinus: (f. 1) *De sacra divinaque arte auri faciendi.*
Cleopatra: (f. 116ᵛ) *De mensuris et ponderibus.*

Escurial, Scorial. Ψ. III. 7; s. XI.

Gregorius Nyssenus: (f. 202) *De hominis opificio* (Des. in cap. 6 ἐδείχθη ἄρα λογικὴ ἡ ψυχή).

Escurial, Scorial. Ψ. IV. 14; s. XV.

Aëtius Amidenus: *Iatricorum libri XVI* (L. I–VI).

Escurial, Scorial. Ω. I. 8; s. XIV.

Aëtius Amidenus: *Iatricorum libri XVI* (Frgm. Π. κατάρρου καὶ κορύζης = l. VIII 57, f. 167 Ald. et π. βηχὸς = l. VIII f. 169 Ald.).
Paulus Aegineta: (f. 1) *Epitomae medicae libri septem medicae libri septem* (Frgm.).
Alexander Trallianus: (f. 1, 15, 20, 22) *Excerpta*.
Aëtius Amidenus: (f. 22ᵛ) *Iatricorum libri XVI* (Frgm. Π. ὀρθοπνοικῶν ἀσθματικῶν τῶν λεγομένων δυσπνοικῶν, ἐκ τῶν Γαλ.).
Asclepiades: (f. 24) *Excerpta varia* (Ἀσθματικόν. Inc. Ἀριστολοχία στρογγύλη. Ex Aetio).
Dioscurides: (f. 24) *Excerpta* (Ἀσθματικόν. Inc. Ἀριστολοχία στρογγύλη).
Paulus Aegineta: (f. 26.) *Epitomae medicae libri septem medicae libri septem* (Frgm.).
Aëtius Amidenus: (f. 31) *Iatricorum libri XVI* (Frgm. Π. τῶν ἐν καρδίᾳ παλμῶν, ἐκ τῶν Γαλ. = l. VIII 64).
Paulus Aegineta: (f. 31ᵛ) *Epitomae medicae libri septem medicae libri septem* (Frgm.).
Aëtius Amidenus: (f. 34ᵛ) *Iatricorum libri XVI* (Frgm. Π. αἵματος ἀναγωγῆς, ἐκ τῶν Γαλ.).
Paulus Aegineta: (f. 42 etc.) *Epitomae medicae libri septem medicae libri septem* (Frgm.).
Alexander Trallianus: (f. 48ᵛ *und öfter*) *Excerpta*.
Aëtius Amidenus: *Iatricorum libri XVI*:
(f. 55) Frgm. Π. τῶν ἐν τῇ τραχείᾳ ἀρτηρίᾳ ἑλκῶν.
(f. 55ᵛ) Frgm. Π. ἐμπυηματικῶν.
(f. 58) Frgm. Π. ἐμπύων καὶ φισιάσεως [sic !].
Abraham: (f. 78ᵛ) *Excerpta* (Στήλη ἐκλίγματος · ἐξελέξατο αὐτὴν ἀβραὰμ ὁ τοῦ Σολομῶντος τῷ ἔχοντι βῆχας κτλ.).

Florenz, Bibl. Mediceo Laurentiana
Firenze, Biblioteca Medicea Laurenziana

Florenz, Bibl. Mediceo Laurentiana, Conventi soppressi 59; s. XIV.

Dioscurides: (f. 1) *De materia medica* (Frgm. ex l. II 1–V 103 = Spr. 167, 10–771, 12).

Florenz, Bibl. Mediceo Laurentiana, Conventi soppressi 627 (Abb. 2728); s. XII.
= Conv. soppr. 627 (*Census*: 68, nr [0284]).

Splenius philosophus: (f. 92ᵛ) *De generatione hominis* (Sine auctoris nomine).

Florenz, Bibl. Mediceo Laurentiana, Laurent. –.
= (?) **plut. 57, 50** (p. 41), **59, 17** (p. 42) and/or **87, 16** (p. 50) below (*Census*: 68, nr [0285]).

Oribasius: *Excerpta varia* (Ἐκ τῶν Ὀρ. ὑγιεινῶν παραγγελμάτων).

Florenz, Bibl. Mediceo Laurentiana, Laurent. plut. 4, 10; s. XI.

Splenius philosophus: (p. 299 b) *De generatione hominis* (Sine auct. nomine).

Florenz, Bibl. Mediceo Laurentiana, Laurent. plut. 7, 2; s. XV.

Nemesius Emesenus: *De natura hominis* (*aus Dresd. 57* [above p. 32] *abgeschr.*).

Florenz, Bibl. Mediceo Laurentiana, Laurent. plut. 7, 35; s. XIV.

Nemesius Emesenus: (f. 196) *De natura hominis.*

Florenz, Bibl. Mediceo Laurentiana, Laurent. plut. 28, 13; s. XIV.

Hermes Trismegistus: (f. 221) *Iatromathematica ad Ammonium Aegyptium.*

Florenz, Bibl. Mediceo Laurentiana, Laurent. plut. 28, 14; s. XIV ex., XIV.

Petosiris: *Epistula ad regem Nechepso* cap. σμα' (Ἑτέρα μέθοδος Πετ. scil. περὶ νόσου ζωῆς καὶ θανάτου).
Hermes Trismegistus: (f. 241) *Methodus ad omne inceptum idonea.*

Florenz, Bibl. Mediceo Laurentiana, Laurent. plut. 28, 33, a. 1542.

Hermes Trismegistus: (f. 246ᵛ) *Canon de decubitu infirmorum* (Inscr. Ἑρμοῦ π. κατακλίσεως. Inc. Ψήφισον τὸ ὄνομα. Expl. ὑγιαίνει).

Florenz, Bibl. Mediceo Laurentiana, Laurent. plut. 28, 34; s. XI.

Hermes Trismegistus: (f. 1) *Iatromathematica ad Ammonium Aegyptium* (»Ab editione Ideleriana paululum differt«).
Pancharius: (f. 16) *Compendium de decubitu infirmorum*.
Petosiris: (f. 21) *Epistula ad regem Nechepso* (Inc. Ἡ δὲ ὑπὸ Πετ. προσαχθεῖσα μεθόδος. Expl. ὁ κίνδυνος ἢ οὔ).
Zenarius: (f. 22ᵛ) *Exordia*.
Petosiris: (f. 61) *Epistula ad regem Nechepso* (Περὶ μηνὸς ἀγαθοῦ καὶ φαύλου. Inc. Οὐδὲ τοῦτο ἄτοπόν σε γνῶναι. Expl. τῶν λοιπῶν ἀστέρων δυνόντων).

Florenz, Bibl. Mediceo Laurentiana, Laurent. plut. 28, 44; s. XV.

Adamantius: (p. 2 b) *De ventis* (Inc. Ἐπειδὴ ἐκ τῶν τῆς γῆς ἀναθυμιάσεων. Expl. καὶ οἰκειότεροι μᾶλλον τοῖς σώμασιν ἡμῶν).

Florenz, Bibl. Mediceo Laurentiana, Laurent. plut. 56, 1; s. XIII–XIV.

Adamantius: (f. 284) *De ventis*.

Florenz, Bibl. Mediceo Laurentiana, Laurent. plut. 56, 21; s. XV.

Nemesius Emesenus: *De natura hominis* (*aus Monac. 419 abgeschr.* [below p. 88]).

Florenz, Bibl. Mediceo Laurentiana, Laurent. plut. 57, 50; s. XVI.
See also **Laurent.** – above (p. 40).

Asclepiades: (p. 557 b) *Praecepta salubria* (Sine auctoris nomine. Expl. ἐκφυγεὶς νόσους).

Florenz, Bibl. Mediceo Laurentiana, Laurent. plut. 58, 24; XIV.

Splenius philosophus: (f. 126) *De generatione hominis* (Sine auctoris nomine).

Florenz, Bibl. Mediceo Laurentiana, Laurent. plut. 59, 14; s. XIII, XV.
Dieses Werk (= Philaretus, *De pulsibus*) *von einer Hand des XIII (!) Saec.*; f. 171ᵛ (= Galenos, *De pulsibus ad Antonium*) *andere Hand*; *sonst* s. XV.

Philaretus: *De pulsibus*.
Stephanus Alexandrinus: (p. 12) *Scholia in Hippocratis praenotiones. Sectiones III*.
Philaretus: (f. 162) *De pulsibus*.

Joannis [Damasceni ?]: (f. 227 b) Hippokrates, *De natura pueri* (Frgm. c. comm. Joannis [Damasceni?]. Ed. Dietz, Scholia in Hipp. et Gal. II 205–235).
Ioannes Alexandrinus (nicht Philoponus): (f. 227 b) *Scholia in Hippocratis librum de natura pueri ab ore Ioannis* (Frgm.).

Florenz, Bibl. Mediceo Laurentiana, Laurent. plut. 59, 17; s. XV.
See also **Laurent.** – above (p. 40).

Asclepiades: (p. 74) *Praecepta salubria* (Sine auctoris nomine).

Florenz, Bibl. Mediceo Laurentiana, Laurent. plut. 74, 1; s. XV.

Erotianus: *Vocum Hippocraticarum conlectio.*
Soranus: (p. 8 b) *Hippocratis genus et vita secundum Soranum.*

Florenz, Bibl. Mediceo Laurentiana, Laurent. plut. 74, 2; s. XI.

Palladius: *De cibo et potione.*
Paulus Aegineta: (p. 1) *Epitomae medicae libri septem medicae libri septem.*
Damnastes: (f. 281[v]) *De curatione puerperarum et infantium* (Frgm.).
Iacobus Psychrestus: (p. 282) *Excerpta* (Emplastrum ἐντατικὸν λεγόμενον γαρέλαιον, ὃ ἐσκεύασεν ἡ λυσία, ἢ ἀρχηγός, ἢ τυφάς. Inc. Στέαρ καμήλου ἀνδριῶντος).
Palladius: (p. 282 b) *De cibo et potione.*

Florenz, Bibl. Mediceo Laurentiana, Laurent. plut. 74, 7; s. IX.

Heliodorus: *Excerpta varia* (Περὶ διαφορᾶς καταρτισμῶν. Cf. Orib. IV 333).
Oribasius:
(p. 89 b) *Medicae collectiones ad Iulianum* (L. XLVI–XLIX).
(p. 89 b) *Excerpta varia* (Ἐκ τῶν Γαλ. περὶ καταγμάτων. Inc. Ἐπειδὴ λέλυται).
Asclepiades: (f. 127) *Excerpta varia* (Ὅτι καὶ διὰ νόσον χρονίαν ἔξαρθροί τινες γίγνονται. Quod diuturno morbo quibusdam articuli prolabuntur. Inc. Ὅτι χωρὶς φανερᾶς. Ex Oribas. IV 243).
Heliodorus: (p. 103) *Excerpta varia* (Περὶ καταγμάτων. De fracturis. Inc. Ἐν πρώτοις. Cf. Orib. IV 154. Ed. A. Cocchius, Veterum medicorum chirurgica p. 90 sq.).
Archigenes: (p. 113) *Excerpta varia* (Περὶ ὑποδραμόντος αἵματος. Inc. Ὑποδρομὴ δὲ αἵματος. Ex Orib. IV 193).
Heliodorus: (p. 113) *Excerpta varia* (Περὶ τερηδονισμοῦ κρανίου. De cranii carie. Inc. Τὴν τοῦ κρανίου. Cf. Orib. IV 187).

Archigenes: (p. 114) *Excerpta varia* (Περὶ τῆς τῶν ῥαφῶν διαστάσεως. Inc. Τοὺς δὲ περισωθησομένους. Ex Orib. IV 197).

Antyllus: (p. 115) *Excerpta* (Περὶ ὑδροκεφάλων. Inc. Τὸ ὑδροκέφαλον. Ex Orib. IV 200).

Heliodorus: *Excerpta varia:*

(p. 116) Περὶ ὀστώδους ἐπιφύσεως. De osse excrescente. Inc. Ὀστώδης ἐπίφυσις. Cf. Orib. IV 204.

(p. 116 b) Περὶ ἀλωπεκίας. De capillis fluentibus. Inc. Τῆς ἀλωπεκίας. Cf. Orib. IV 207.

Oribasius: (p. 117) *Excerpta varia* (Ἐκ τῶν Γαλ. περὶ ἐξαρθρημάτων. Inc. Τῶν ἐξαρθρημάτων).

Archigenes: (p. 127) *Excerpta varia* (Περὶ τῶν ἀφαιρεθησομένων μερῶν. Ex Orib. IV 244. *Vgl.* Harles, Anall. histor.-medica de Archigene et de Apolloniis medicis etc. Lips. 1816).

Heliodorus: *Excerpta varia:*

(p. 128) Περὶ ἀκρωτηριασμοῦ. De mutilatione. Cf. Orib. IV 247.

(p. 128 b) Περὶ τῶν κατὰ τοὺς δακτύλους συμβαινόντων. De iis quae digitis accidunt. Inc. Ἐξαδακτύλοι γίνονται. Cf. Orib. IV 249.

Oribasius: *Excerpta varia*:

(p. 129) Ἐκ τοῦ Ἡρακλᾶ πῶς πλέκεται βρόχος ὁ ἐρτός.

(p. 129 b) Ἐκ τῶν Γαλ. περὶ ἐπιδέσμων.

Heliodorus: *Excerpta varia*:

(p. 136 b) Περὶ ἐπιδέσμων. Cf. Orib. IV 281.

(p. 140 b) Μεταγωγεύς. Adducens. Cf. Orib. IV 297.

(p. 141) Κράτημα. Retinaculum. Cf. Orib. IV 299.

(p. 141 b) Χειλοφύλαξ. Custos labiorum. Cf. Orib. IV 301.

Oribasius: (p. 148 b) *Excerpta varia* (Ἐκ τῶν Ἡλιοδώρου περὶ διαφορᾶς καταρτισμῶν).

Heliodorus: (p. 154 b) *Excerpta varia* (Νειλέως πλινθίον. Cf. Orib. IV 357).

Rufus: (p. 173) *Excerpta varia* (Ἐκ τῶν Ῥούφου τὸ Ἱπποκράτους βάθρον. Inc. Ὁ θαυμασιώτατος Ἱπποκράτης. *Aus* Oribas. IV p. 432).

Apollonius Citiensis: (p. 179 b) *Commentarius in Hippocratis de articulis, libri III.*

Soranus:

(p. 224 b) *De signis fracturarum.*

(p. 227) *De fasciis* (*27 Blätter*).

Paulus Aegineta: *Epitomae medicae libri septem medicae libri septem*:

(p. 239 b) Frgm. Libri VII. capp. 89–112.

(p. 252 b) Frgm. Libri VI. cap. 42.

Rufus:

(p. 275) *De corporis humani appellationibus.*

(p. 283 b) *De ossibus.*
Palladius: (p. 299 b) *Scholia in Hippocratis de facturis.*

Florenz, Bibl. Mediceo Laurentiana, Laurent. plut. 74, 10; s. XIV.

Theophilus: *De urinis*:
(p. 15) De urinarum coloribus.
(p. 18 b) Inc. Τὴν π. τῶν οὔρων.
Dioscurides: (p. 27) *De facile parabilibus tam simplicibus quam compositis medicamentis libri II.*
Alexander Trallianus: (p. 86) *Therapeutica. Libri XII.*

Florenz, Bibl. Mediceo Laurentiana, Laurent. plut. 74, 11; s. XIII.

Theophilus:
(p. 1) *Commentarius in Hippocratis aphorismos* (Initio mutilus).
(p. 131 b) *De urinis* (Inc. Οὖρόν ἐστι τὸ περιήθημα).
Severianus: (p. 150) *Definitiones* (Inc. Τί Θεὸς ὄνομα κυρίως. Expl. Τί φρὴν κτέ.).
Palladius:
(p. 200–242^{v}) *In Galeni librum de sectis scholia* (Expl. mutil.).
(f. 211^{v}) *Stephani philosophi vel Palladii synopsis de febribus* (Scholia in Galeni de febrium differentiis. *Vgl.* [Vatic.] Palat. 297 [below p. 151]).

Florenz, Bibl. Mediceo Laurentiana, Laurent. plut. 74, 13; s. XV.

Soranus: (p. 3) *Hippocratis genus et vita secundum Soranum.*
Ioannes Zacharias Actuarius: (p. 88) *De urinis libri VII.*
Hypatus: (p. 301 b) *Interpretatio partium corporis.*

Florenz, Bibl. Mediceo Laurentiana, Laurent. plut. 74, 15; s. XIV.

Oribasius: (p. 1) *Conspectus ad Eustathium filium. Libri II.*

Florenz, Bibl. Mediceo Laurentiana, Laurent. plut. 74, 17; s. XII.

Oribasius:
(f. 1) *Medicae collectiones ad Iulianum* (Inc. Ἡ ὠμαία κατ' ἀγκῶνα).
(p. 1) *Conspectus ad Eustathium filium. Libri II.*
Paulus Aegineta: (p. 106 b) *Epitomae medicae libri septem* (Frgm. Libri I. capp. 1–30).
Dioscurides: (p. 112) *De materia medica* (Liber V qui des. imperfecte. »Hic codex pars est codicis [Venet.] Marc. 273 [below p. 170].« Wellmann).

Florenz, Bibl. Mediceo Laurentiana, Laurent. plut. 74, 20; s. XV.

Dioscurides: (p. 1) *De facile parabilibus tam simplicibus quam compositis medicamentis libri II.*

Florenz, Bibl. Mediceo Laurentiana, Laurent. plut. 74, 21; s. XV.

Paulus Aegineta:
(p. 1) *Epitomae medicae libri septem* (Frgm. Libri VI. capp. 89–122).
(p. 36 b) *Epitomae medicae libri septem* (Frgm. L. V 1. part. 2. 28. 29. 7. 11. L. VII 1. part. 17. 3).
(p. 46) *Epitomae medicae libri septem* (Frgm. »X capp. forte eiusdem Pauli Aeg.«).

Florenz, Bibl. Mediceo Laurentiana, Laurent. plut. 74, 23; s. XIV.

Dioscurides:
(p. 1) *De materia medica* (Libri IX).
(f. 183v) *De venenis eorumque praecautione et medicatione.*
(f. 190v) *De iis, quae virus eiaculantur, animalibus libellus, in quo et de rabioso cane* (Tribus libris dispos.).
Paulus Aegineta:
(f. 200v) *De succedaneis, ex Galeno.*
(f. 204) *De mensuris et ponderibus.*
Africanus: (p. 204) *Ex Africani Cestis cestum XIII cap. 22: De purgantibus simplicibus* (Inc. Κυκλωμένου χυλῷ. Expl. μιχθεὶς καὶ ποθείς).
Paulus Aegineta: (p. 204) *Epitomae medicae libri septem* (Frgm. L. VII 26 extr. Inc. Ὁ σταθμὸς βάρει).

Florenz, Bibl. Mediceo Laurentiana, Laurent. plut. 74, 24, s. XV.

Paulus Aegineta: (p. 1) *Epitomae medicae libri septem* (Liber VI).

Florenz, Bibl. Mediceo Laurentiana, Laurent. plut. 74, 26; s. XIV (»L. VI saec. XV scriptus est«).

Paulus Aegineta: (p. 1) *Epitomae medicae libri septem* (L. V–VII. »L. VI saec. xv scriptus est«).

Florenz, Bibl. Mediceo Laurentiana, Laurent. plut. 74, 27; s. XIV.

Paulus Aegineta: (p. 1) *Epitomae medicae libri septem.*

Florenz, Bibl. Mediceo Laurentiana, Laurent. plut. 74, 29; s. XI.

Paulus Aegineta: (p. 1) *Epitomae medicae libri septem* (L. I–IV. L. V 22. 23. 26. 3).

Florenz, Bibl. Mediceo Laurentiana, Laurent. plut. 74, 31; x. XIV.

Paulus Aegineta: (p. 1) *Epitomae medicae libri septem* (L. I–VII 25).
Theophilus:
(p. 34) *De pulsibus*.
(p. 34) *De alvi excrementis*.

Florenz, Bibl. Mediceo Laurentiana, Laurent. plut. 75, 2; s. XIV.

Aëtius Amidenus: (p. 1) *Iatricorum libri XVI* (L. IX–XV).

Florenz, Bibl. Mediceo Laurentiana, Laurent. plut. 75, 3; s. XII.

Metrodora: (f. 4–33) *De mulierum morbis uteri* (*Vgl.* Daremb. Orib. I p. XXV).
Marcianus: (p. 263) *Medicamentum ad nervos laxandos idoneum*.

Florenz, Bibl. Mediceo Laurentiana, Laurent. plut. 75, 4; s. XV.

Paulus Aegineta: (p. 235) *De succedaneis, ex Galeno*.

Florenz, Bibl. Mediceo Laurentiana, Laurent. plut. 75, 5; s. XIV.
»Laurent. 75, 5 + 75, 20 bilden Bd. I, 75, 18 + 75, 7 den II. Bd. derselben Aëtiushandschrift des XIV. Jahrhunderts.« M. W.

Aëtius Amidenus: *Iatricorum libri XVI*:
(p. 1) L. VI–VIII.; *vgl.* Olivieri, L'oftalmologia di Aetios nel cod. Laur. 75, 5 in: Studi italiani XII p. 261 ff.
(p. 151 b) Ex l. II et III.

Florenz, Bibl. Mediceo Laurentiana, Laurent. plut. 75, 6; s. XIV.

Diodorus: (f. 127) *De mensuris et ponderibus*.

Florenz, Bibl. Mediceo Laurentiana, Laurent. plut. 75, 7; s. XIV.
»Laurent. 75, 5 + 75, 20 bilden Bd. I, 75, 18 + 75, 7 den II. Bd. derselben Aëtiushandschrift des XIV. Jahrhunderts.« M. W.

Aëtius Amidenus: (p. 1) *Iatricorum libri XVI* (L. XIII–XVI).
Rufus:
(p. 214) *Conspectus de pulsibus* (*Vorangeht:* Ἐγὼ προσέθηκα τοῦτο τὸ π.

σφυγμῶν μονόβιβλον · τὸ γὰρ σύνταγμα οὐκ εἶχε · νομίζω δὲ αὐτὸ μὴ εἶναι Γαληνοῦ, ἀλλὰ Ῥούφου τοῦ Ἐφεσίου).

(p. 219) *De medicamentis purgantibus* (Inc. Οὔτε πάντας τοὺς ὅπως).

Antyllus: *Excerpta*:

(p. 224) Διαιτητικά. Ex libro II. de victus ratione. Inc. Τῶν καθαιρόντων τὰ μέν. Ed. C. F. Wolz, Antylli veteris chirurgi quae ap. Orib. libro 44. 45 et 50 leguntur. Diss. inaug. Jen. 1842.

(p. 225) Περὶ κλυσμῶν, ὅτι διὰ τρεῖς αἰτίας παραλαμβάνονται. Inc. Παραλαμβάνονται οἱ κλυσμοί. »Antyllo tribuit Bandini III p. 151«.

Severus: (p. 225 b) *De instrumentis infusoriis seu clysteribus ad Timotheum*.

Florenz, Bibl. Mediceo Laurentiana, Laurent. plut. 75, 8; s. XV.

Aëtius Amidenus: *Excerpta varia*:

(p. 1) Διάγνωσις οὔρου.

(p. 3) Ἀκριβεστάτη σύνοψις περὶ οὔρων ἐκ τῆς ἰατρικῆς τέχνης τῶν Περσῶν. Inc. Τὸ οὖρον μέχρι καὶ τῆς.

(p. 3 b) Περὶ τῆς ἐκ σφυγμῶν σημειώσεως excerptum brevissimum.

Dioscurides: (p. 4) *Liber agens de experientia medica, de simplicibus et compositis medicamentis, ordine literarum digestus* (Frgm. litteram A non excedens).

Ioannes Zacharias Actuarius: (p. 222) *De methodo medendi Libri VI.*

Dioscurides: (p. 438) *Excerpta* (Quaedam medica βοηθήματα. Inc. Χολιάνδρου κόκκους. Ad D. pertinere susp. Bandini III 153).

Diocles: (p. 454 b) *Ad Antigonum regem epistula de tuenda valetitudine.*

Florenz, Bibl. Mediceo Laurentiana, Laurent. plut. 75, 9; s. XV.

Ioannes Zacharias Actuarius:

(p. 5) *De urinis libri VII.*

(p. 114) *De spiritu animali libri II.*

Paulus Aegineta: (p. 460) *De succedaneis, ex Galeno.*

Florenz, Bibl. Mediceo Laurentiana, Laurent. plut. 75, 10; s. XV.

Ioannes Archiatrus: (f. 32) *Variorum morborum curatio* (Τοῦ σοφωτάτου Ἀριστοτέλους λόγοι καὶ προοίμια, κυρίου Ἰωάννου ἀρχιάτρου καὶ μαθητοῦ αὐτοῦ, περιέχων συνοπτικῶς πάντων τῶν παθῶν καὶ τῶν ἀδήλων τὰς θεραπείας. Inc. Πρὸς ὀξὺν πόνον κεφαλῆς. Ἔπαρον ἀγριαγκουρέας σπόρον. Expl. θέτ' ἐς τὸ μέτωπον).

Aëtius Amidenus:

(f. 51–52^{v}) *Excerpta varia* (»Excerpte aus B. XIII.« M. W.).

(p. 55) *Iatricorum libri XVI* (L. IX cap. extr.-XII 69).

(f. 55–134) *Iatricorum libri XVI* (M.W.)
(f. 329) *Excerpta varia* (Ἐκ τῶν Ἀετίου περὶ τῶν ἐν τοῖς σπλάγχνοις ἐρυσιπελάτων διαθέσεων κτλ. »Sind Excerpte aus B. XII«. M. W.).

Florenz, Bibl. Mediceo Laurentiana, Laurent. plut. 75, 11; s. XV.

Ioannes Zacharias Actuarius:
(p. 1) *De urinis libri VII* (Libri XI).
(p. 82) *De spiritu animali libri II.*
(p. 116 b) *De methodo medendi Libri VI.*
(p. 286) *De succedaneis, ex Galeno.*

Florenz, Bibl. Mediceo Laurentiana, Laurent. plut. 75, 12; s. XV.

Aëtius Amidenus: (p. 1) *Iatricorum libri XVI* (L. I–III).

Florenz, Bibl. Mediceo Laurentiana, Laurent. plut. 75, 13; s. XV.

Aëtius Amidenus: (p. 1) *Iatricorum libri XVI* (L. XIV–XVI).
Alexander Aphrodisiensis: (p. 121) *Problematum physicorum et medicorum eclogae. Libri V* (Libri I et II).

Florenz, Bibl. Mediceo Laurentiana, Laurent. plut. 75, 14; s. XV.

Alexander Aphrodisiensis: (p. 1) *De febribus.*

Florenz, Bibl. Mediceo Laurentiana, Laurent. plut. 75, 15; s. XV.

Aretaeus:
(p. 1) *De causis et signis acutorum morborum libri II* (L. I c. 1–4 perierunt).
(f. 15) *De causis et signis diuturnorum morborum libri II.*
(p. 40) *De curatione acutorum morborum libri II.*
(p. 63) *De curatione diuturnorum morborum libri II.*

Florenz, Bibl. Mediceo Laurentiana, Laurent. plut. 75, 16; s. XV.

Beniaminus: (p. 3) *Medicamenta purgantia omne cerebri ac stomachi excrementum.*
Ioannes Zacharias Actuarius:
(p. 4) *De urinis libri VII.*
(p. 105) *De spiritu animali libri II.*
(p. 192 b) *De methodo medendi Libri VI.*
(p. 383 b) *De succedaneis, ex Galeno.*

Florenz, Bibl. Mediceo Laurentiana, Laurent. plut. 75, 18; s. XIV.
»Laurent. 75, 5 + 75, 20 bilden Bd. I, 75, 18 + 75, 7 den II. Bd. derselben Aëtiushandschrift des XIV. Jahrhunderts.« M. W.

Aëtius Amidenus: (p. 1) *Iatricorum libri XVI* (L. IX–XIII).

Florenz, Bibl. Mediceo Laurentiana, Laurent. plut. 75, 19; s. XIV.

Coeranus: (p. 5) *De arte recuratoria* (Frgm.).
Meletius monachus: (p. 8 b) *De natura hominis*.
Theophilus: (p. 82 b) *Therapeutica Theophili, quam ipse ex variis libris valetudinariis collegit*.

Florenz, Bibl. Mediceo Laurentiana, Laurent. plut. 75, 20; s. XIV.
»Laurent. 75, 5 + 75, 20 bilden Bd. I, 75, 18 + 75, 7 den II. Bd. derselben Aëtiushandschrift des XIV. Jahrhunderts.« M. W.

Aëtius Amidenus: (p. 1) *Iatricorum libri XVI* (L. I–V).

Florenz, Bibl. Mediceo Laurentiana, Laurent. plut. 75, 21; s. XIII.

Aëtius Amidenus: (p. 1) *Iatricorum libri XVI* (L. IX–XVI).
Palladius: (p. 251) *Scholia in Hippocratis de popularibus morbis librum sextum, sectiones VIII* (Frgm. »Sextae et septimae sectionis fragmentum« = Dietz II p. 161, 21–171, 34. 177, 18–198, 19).

Florenz, Bibl. Mediceo Laurentiana, Laurent. plut. 75, 22; s. XV.

Palladius: (p. 1) *Scholia in Hippocratis de popularibus morbis librum sextum, sectiones VIII*.

Florenz, Bibl. Mediceo Laurentiana, Laurent. plut. 86, 6; s. XII.

Nemesius Emesenus: (f. 1) *De natura hominis* (Ἀδαμαντίωνος τοῦ καὶ Νεμεσίου).

Florenz, Bibl. Mediceo Laurentiana, Laurent. plut. 86, 14; s. XV.

Petosiris:
(f. 95ᵛ) *Excerpta* (Κύκλος Πετοσίρι⟨δος⟩).
(f. 96) *Epistula ad regem Nechepso* (Inc. Περὶ ἑνὸς ἑκάστου. Expl. *wie im* plut. 28, 34 [see p. 41). Ed. Rieß *a. a. O. p.* 385).

Florenz, Bibl. Mediceo Laurentiana, Laurent. plut. 86, 16; a. 1492.

Synesius: *Ad Dioscorum, scholia in librum Democriti*.

Democritus: (sect. 35) *Liber V ad Leucippum.*

Florenz, Bibl. Mediceo Laurentiana, Laurent. plut. 86, 20; s. XV.

Stephanus Atheniensis: (f. 64) *De febrium differentiis ex ore Theophili.*
Theophilus: (f. 64) *Epitome librorum Galeni de febrium differentiis.*

Florenz, Bibl. Mediceo Laurentiana, Laurent. plut. 87, 16; s. XIII.
See also **Laurent.** – above (p. 40).

Asclepiades: (p. 14) *Praecepta salubria* (Sine auctoris nomine. Expl. λατρόφωνος εὑρέθη).

Florenz, Bibl. Mediceo Laurentiana, Laurent. App., 2; s. XV.
= Antinori 101 (*Census*: 80, nr [0372]).

Mercurius monachus: (f. 83^{v}) *De pulsibus* (»Περὶ σφυγμῶν. Sunt nr. 25–28 tractatus Mercurio tributi, Ideler II p. 256, sed post n. 25 inseruntur Κράτησον τὸν σφυγμὸν, καὶ εἰ μὲν ῥίπτει ὅλον ἔξω ἀραιά, ἕως ἡμέρας τρεῖς ἐστιν ἡ ζωὴ αὐτοῦ«).
Dioscurides: (f. 236^{v}) *De mensuris et ponderibus* (»Fere eadem quae apud Hu. p. 240, 1–241, 4. 242, 12–244, 8«).
Heliodorus: (f. 240) *De mensuris et ponderibus* (Expl. ὀβολοὺς ξε').
Paulus Aegineta: (f. 245) *De succedaneis, ex Galeno.*
Hermes Trismegistus: (f. 256^{v}) *Excerpta varia* (Ἀντίδοτος αἰγυπτιακή. Inc. Πρὸς ποδαλγικούς. Expl. οὐκ ἀποτυγχάνει).
Beniaminus, Andromachus, Paulus Aegineta: (f. 272^{v}) *Excerpta.*
Paulus Aegineta:
(f. 273^{v}) *Excerpta.*
(f. 339) εἰς κοιλιοστόμαχον.
Alexander Trallianus: (f. 323) *Epistula de lumbricis.*
Paulus Aegineta: *Excerpta*:
(f. 327^{v}) πρὸς ἑλμίνθας.
(f. 328) Ἐκ τοῦ Παύλου.
Alexander Trallianus: (f. 328^{v}, 332, 338) *Excerpta varia.*
Paulus Aegineta: *Excerpta*:
(f. 339^{v}) π. λυγμοῦ.
(f. 340) πρὸς τὸ ποιῆσαι ὄρεξιν.
Democritus: (f. 340^{v}) *Excerpta* (Πρὸς ἔμετον στομάχου).
Theodorus: *Excerpta*:
(f. 342^{v}) Εἰς ἔμφραξιν στομάχου δοθὲν παρὰ Θεοδώρου τῶν Μαγγάνων).
(f. 343) Πρόσταξις στομαχικὴ τοῦ ξενῶνος τῶν Μαγγάνων.

Stephanus Ἀρχιατρὸς τῶν Μαγγάνων: (f. 343) *Epistula* (Ἐπιστολὴ ἀπὸ Θεσσαλονίκης παρὰ Στεφάνου ἀρχιιατροῦ τῶν Μεγγάνων [sic] etc.).
Alexander Trallianus: (f. 345v, 346) *Excerpta varia.*
Paulus Aegineta: (f. 349v) *Excerpta* (π. ἥπατος).
Abraham: (f. 353v) *Excerpta* (Τοῦ Σαρακηνοῦ τοῦ Ἀβράμη καὶ Ἀκταρίου τῶν Μαγγάνων καὶ βασιλικοῦ ἀρχιατροῦ βοήθημα καθαρτικὸν ἐπί τε ἡπατικῶν ἰκτερικῶν καὶ σπληνικῶν καὶ ἰσχιαδικῶν. Inc. Ἀλι λέκχ · ἤγουν χρυσοβάλανον).
Eustathius: (f. 355) *Excerpta* (Inc. Ἤκουσα καγώ Εὐστάθιος ὁ εὐτελὴς ἰατρός).
Democritus: (f. 356) *Excerpta* (Παύλου γενικοῦ καὶ Δημοκρίτου περὶ πόνων ἰσχίου).
Paulus Aegineta: *Excerpta*:
(f. 356) Παύλ. καὶ Δημοκρίτου π. πόνων ἰσχίου.
(f. 358) ἐπὶ ἰσχιδιακῶν.
Eleutherus: (f. 358) *Excerpta* (Ἐπὶ ἰσχιαδκικῶν).
Democritus: (f. 359) *Excerpta* (Περὶ φλεγμονῆς γαργαρεῶνος. Inc. Γαργαρεὼν ἐστι ἡ λεγομένη παρά).
Paulus Aegineta: (f. 359) *Excerpta* (π. κιονίδος).
Hermes Trismegistus: (f. 361) *Excerpta varia* (Ἀντίδοτος ἀρθρητική, ποδαλγικὴ καὶ νεφριτική. Inc. Ποδαλγικὴ ἀντίδοτος ἐκ τῶν Ἡφαίστου ἀδύτων ἐν Μεμφίδι).

Florenz, bibl. naz. [Magliabecchiana] / Magliabech.
Now Firenze, Biblioteca nazionale Magliabechiana

Florenz, bibl. naz. [Magliabecchiana], II.III.304; s. XVI.
Now *Magliabechianus* 30 (*Census*: 80, nr [0373]).

Eutecnius: *Paraphrasis in Nicandri Theriaca* (Inc. Τῶν ἑρπετῶν θηρίων ὁπόσα ἐστίν. Expl. οὗτός ποτε γένηται τοῦ πλῆξαι).

Florenz, Magliabech. 44; s. XII.

Paulus Aegineta: (f. 2) *De succedaneis, ex Galeno.*

Florenz, Bibl. Riccardiana
Firenze, Biblioteca Riccardiana

Florenz, Bibl. Riccardiana, Riccard. 10 (K I 12); a. 1583.
Now Riccard. 10 (*Census*: 81, nr [0377]).

Alexander Trallianus: (f. 67) *Therapeutica. Libri XII.*

Florenz, Bibl. Riccardiana, Riccard. 31 (K II 4); s. XIV.
Now Riccard. 31 (*Census*: 81, nr [0379]).

Ioannes Zacharias Actuarius: (f. 275) *De spiritu animali libri II* (»Titulus hic prolatus ab usitato valde discrepat«).

Florenz, Bibl. Riccardiana, Riccard. 71 (K II 16); a. 1428.
Now Riccard. 71 (*Census*: 81, nr [0382]).

Paulus Aegineta: (f. 108) *De succedaneis, ex Galeno.*

Florenz, Bibl. Riccardiana, Riccard. 91 (K II 7); s. XV.
Now Riccard. 91 (*Census*: 81, nr [0383]).

Dioscurides: *De facile parabilibus tam simplicibus quam compositis medicamentis libri II.*

Genua

Genua, Bibl. della Missione urbana, 17; s. IX ex. – X.
= Genova, Biblioteca Franzoniana, Urbani 17 (*Census*: 84, nr [0386]).

Gregorius Nyssenus: (f. 213) *De hominis opificio.*

Glasgow

Glasgow, Hunterian Museum, V.5.11; s. XV.
Now Glasgow, Glasgow University Library, Special Collections Department, Ms Hunter 271 (U.5.11) (*Census*: 84, nr [0387]).

Ioannes Zacharias Actuarius: (f. 1) *De spiritu animali libri II.*

Göttingen, Univ.-Bibl.
Now Göttingen, Niedersachsische Staats- und Universitätsbibliothek

Göttingen, Univ.-Bibl., Hist. nat., 5; s. XVII.
Now 4° Cod. Ms. hist. nat. 5 (*Census*: 84, nr [0390]).

Theophilus: *Commentarius in Hippocratis aphorismos.*

Göttingen, Univ.-Bibl., Hist. nat., 6; a. 1670.
Now 8° Cod. Ms. hist. nat. 6 (*Census*: 84, nr [0391]).

Dioscurides: *Excerpta* (Simplicium facultates medicae ex antiquis, opera et stud. G. H. Welsch).

Göttingen, Univ.-Bibl., Hist. nat., 90; a. 1598.
Now 2° Cod. Ms. hist. nat. 90 (*Census*: 84, nr [0392]).

Dioscurides: *De materia medica* (impr. a. 1598 c. nott. mss. Ioh. Grammi [1685–1749]).

Hamburg

Hamburg, nr. – (*Vgl.* Fabricius bibl. gr. IX. p. 454–474).
Now Staats- und Universitätsbibliothek Hamburg «Carl von Ossietzky», philol. 313 (*Census*: 87, nr [0397]).
Same as **Hamburgens. 200** below.

Xenocrates: *De alimento ex aquatilibus.*

Hamburg, Stadtbibliothek, Hamburgens. 200.
Now Staats- und Universitätsbibliothek Hamburg «Carl von Ossietzky», philol. 313 (*Census*: 87, nr [0397]).
Same as above.

Xenocrates: (f. 21–27) *De alimento ex aquatilibus* (in den Philologica Hamburgensia, Hambg. 1905 = philol. 313; s. XVII. f. 21–27.).

Heidelberg, Bibl. Univ.
Now Heidelberg, Universitätsbibliothek

Heidelberg, Bibl. Univ., 375; s. XIV.
= Cod. Pal. graec. 375 (*Census*: 89, nr [0401]).

Oribasius: (nr 3) *Medicae collectiones ad Iulianum* (Liber XXIV, init. et fine mutil.).

Holkham

Holkham, Bibl. des Gr. Leicester, 283; s. XVI.
Now Oxford, Bodleian Library, MS. Holkham Gr. 108 (*Census*: 89, nr [0404]).
See also **Padua, Bibl. S. Joannis in Viridario, ad dextr. plut. 16** below (p. 101).

Aëtius Amidenus: (f. 1) *Iatricorum libri XVI* (L. I–VIII).

Holkham, Bibl. des Gr. Leicester, 289; s. XII.
Now Oxford, Bodleian Library, MS. Holkham Gr. 113 (*Census*: 89–90, nr [0405]).

Epiphanius: (f. 175) *De mensuris et ponderibus* (Expl. λίτραν μίαν καὶ Γο Γο η').

Holkham, Bibl. des Gr. Leicester, 293; s. XV.
Now Oxford, Bodleian Library, MS. Holkham Gr. 106 (*Census*: 90, nr [0406]).

Synesius: (f. 1) *De insomniis* (c. comm.).

Jena, Universitätsbibliothek. Now Thüringer Universitäts- und Landesbibliothek

Jena, Universitätsbibliothek, Jenens.
= Ms. Bos. f. 1 (*Census*: 91, nr [0407]).

Epiphanius: *De mensuris et ponderibus II.*

Jerusalem, Bibl. d. hl. Grabes Now at Αθήνα, Εθνική Βιβλιοθήκη της Ελλάδος ΕΒΕ, Μετόχιον Παναγίου Τάφου–ΜΠΤ

Jerusalem, Bibl. d. hl. Grabes, 38; s. XVII.
Now ΜΠΤ 83 (*Census*: 92, nr [0409]).

Rufus: (nr 2) *De vesicae renumque affectibus.*

Jerusalem, Bibl. d. hl. Grabes, 273; s. X.
Now ΜΠΤ 273 (*Census*: 92, nr [0413] and p. 15).

Nemesius Emesenus: (f. 182 b) *De natura hominis.*

Jerusalem, Bibl. d. hl. Grabes, 304; a. 1615.
Now ΜΠΤ 304 (*Census*: 92, nr [0414] and p. 15).

Meletius monachus: (f. 103) *De natura hominis.*

Jerusalem, Bibl. d. hl. Grabes, 357; s. XVI.
Now ΜΠΤ 357 (*Census*: 92, nr [0415] and p. 15).

Meletius monachus: (f. 304) *De natura hominis.*

Jerusalem, Bibl. d. hl. Grabes, 405; a. 1717.
Now ΜΠΤ 405 (*Census*: 92, nr [0417]).

Nemesius Emesenus: (f. 124) *De natura hominis.*

Jerusalem, Bibl. Mar-Saba
Ιερουσαλήμ, Πατριαρχείο, Ιερά Μονή Αγίου Σάββα

Jerusalem, Bibl. Mar-Saba, 366; s. –.
= Ιερά Μονή Αγίου Σάββα, 366 (*Census*: 93, nr [0420]).

Gregorius Nyssenus: (f. 101) *De hominis opificio.*

Jerusalem, Bibl. Mar-Saba, 432; a. 1662.
= Ιερά Μονή Αγίου Σάββα, 432 (*Census*: 93, nr [0421]).

Hippokrates, **Galenos**, **Meletius monachus**: (f. 1) *Jatrosophium* (Ἰατροσόφιον … Γαλ. Ἱππ. καὶ Μελετίου).

Jerusalem, Bibl. patriarch.
Ιερουσαλήμ, Πατριαρχείο, Πανάγιος Τάφος

Jerusalem, Bibl. patriarch., 15; s. XI.
= Πανάγιος Τάφος, 15 (*Census*: 94, nr [0424]).

Nemesius Emesenus: (f. 137 [*hinter*]) *De natura hominis.*

Jerusalem, Bibl. patriarch., 108; s. XIII.
= Πανάγιος Τάφος, 108 (*Census*: 94, nr [0426]).

Alexander Aphrodisiensis: (f. 80 B) *Problematum physicorum et medicorum eclogae. Libri V* (Frgm.).

Jerusalem, Bibl. patriarch., 148; s. XVI.
= Πανάγιος Τάφος, 148 (*Census*: 94, nr [0427]).

Gregorius Theologus: (f. 56) *Alatium.*
Stephanus Atheniensis: (f. 56^{v}) *Dioscoridis et Stephani Atheniensis de pharmacis ordine literarum* (Frgm.).

Jerusalem, Bibl. patriarch., 203; s. XIX.
= Πανάγιος Τάφος, 203 (*Census*: 94, nr [0428]).

Meletius monachus: (f. 189) *De natura hominis.*

Jerusalem, Bibl. patriarch., 273; s. XVIII.
= Πανάγιος Τάφος, 273 (*Census*: 94, nr [0429]).

Aëtius Amidenus: (f. 1) *Excerpta varia* (Χολῆς ξανθῆς καθαρτικόν. Inc. Ἀλόη τὸ μὲν ὅλον).
Paulus Aegineta: (p. 107) *Epitomae medicae libri septem* (L. III 15).
Rufus: (f. 108) *Excerpta varia* (Ἡ Ῥούφου ἱερά).

Jerusalem, Bibl. patriarch., 339; s.XVI.
= Πανάγιος Τάφος, 339 (*Census*: 94, nr [0430]).

Paulus Aegineta: (f. 64^{v}) *De succedaneis, ex Galeno.*

Jerusalem, Bibl. patriarch., 470; s. XVIII.
= Πανάγιος Τάφος, 470 (*Census*: 95, nr [0432]).

Meletius monachus: (f. 1) *De natura hominis.*

Jerusalem, Bibl. patriarch., 511; XVIII.XIX.
= Πανάγιος Τάφος, 511 (*Census*: 95, nr [0433]).

Meletius monachus: (nr 2) *De natura hominis.*

Karlsruhe, Großherzogl. Hof. u. Landesbibliothek
Now Badische Landesbibliothek Karlsruhe

Karlsruhe, Großherzogl. Hof. u. Landesbibliothek, 451; s. XVI.
Now K 451 (*Census*: 95, nr [0435]).

Nemesius Emesenus: (f. 1–128) *De natura hominis* (*aus Monac. 419* [p. 88] *abgeschr.*).

Kopenhagen, Bibl. Univ.
Now København, Kongelige Bibliotek

Kopenhagen, Bibl. Univ., e donatione variorum 4° 277; s. XV–XVI.
Now Add. 277 4° (*Census*: 102, nr [0449]).

Dioscurides: (f. 5) *De facile parabilibus tam simplicibus quam compositis medicamentis libri II.*

Kopenhagen, Bibl. Univ., e donatione variorum fol. 29; s. XV–XVI.
Now e don. var. 29, 2° (*Census*: 102, nr [0451]).
See also **Padua, Bibl. Joann. Rhodii** below (p. 101).

Stephanus Atheniensis: *Enarratio Galeni de methodo medendi ad Glauconem librorum.*

Kopenhagen, Königl. Bibliothek.
Now København, Det Kongelige Bibliotek

Kopenhagen, Königl. Bibliothek, Hauniens. ant. fund. reg. 224; s. XVI.
Now GkS 224, 2° (*Census*: 102, nr [0445]).

Soranus: *Hippocratis genus et vita secundum Soranum.*

Krakau, Bibl. Univ. Jagellon.
Now Kraków, Biblioteca Jagiellońska, Uniwersytet Jagiellońska w Krakowie

Krakau, Bibl. Univ. Jagellon., 2526 FF VI 5; s. XV.
Now Biblioteca Jagiellońska, Uniwersytet Jagiellońska w Krakowie, BJ 2526 (*Census*: 103, nr [0452]).

Meletius monachus: (f. 1) *De natura hominis* (Inc. Τὰ περὶ τῆς τοῦ ἀνθρώπου κατασκευῆς. Expl. καὶ ἔξωθεν ἐμπλάσας ἐπιτίθει).
Theophilus: (f. 86ᵛ) *De urinis.*
Petosiris: (f. 98) *Epistula ad regem Nechepso* (Inc. Ἐπειδὴ βεβάρηταί σου. Expl. ἐν τῷ ὑπογείῳ ἀποθνήσκει. *Vgl.* Rieß *a. a. O. p.* 384 [= Rieß, Nechepsonis et Petosiridis fragmenta magica. Philol. Suppl. VI p. 325–394]).
Ioannes Episcopus Prisdianensis: (f. 99) *Collectanea de urinis* (Expl. ἢ ὑπὸ πλήθους τοῦ χυμοῦ).

Leipzig

Leipzig, Bibl. senat., 391; s. XVIII.
Now Universitätsbibliothek Rep. I 36aa (*Census*: 108, nr [0471]).

Aëtius Amidenus: *Iatricorum libri XVI* (L. IX–XVI. *Ist der Codex Boerhaaves. Apogr. des Vindob. med. 6* [below p. 178] *nach Zervos*).

Leipzig, Universitätsbibliothek
Now Leipzig, Universitätsbibliothek «Bibliotheca Albertina»

Leipzig, Universitätsbibliothek, 59; s. XIX.
= Cod. graec. 59 (*Census*: 107, nr [0463]).

Oribasius: (nr 1) *Medicae collectiones ad Iulianum* (L. XLIII).
Apollonius Citiensis: (nr 2) *Commentarius in Hippocratis de articulis, libri III* (conscr. a Fr. del Furia Florentino et a K. G. Kuehnio).

Leipzig, Universitätsbibliothek, 60; a. 1786. 87.
= Cod. graec. 60 (*Census*: 107, nr [0464]).

Ioannes Zacharias Actuarius: *De methodo medendi libri VI.*

Leipzig, Universitätsbibliothek, 62; s. XIX.
= Cod. graec. 62 (*Census*: 107, nr [0466]).

Paulus Aegineta: *Epitomae medicae libri septem* (»Paul. Aeg. ex editione Aldina descriptus cum coniecturis Salmasii«).

Leipzig, Universitätsbibliothek, 63 (ol. 1109?); s. XVI.
= Cod. graec. 63 (*Census*: 107, nr [0467]).

Aretaeus:
(f. 1) *De causis et signis acutorum morborum libri II.*
(f. 14) *De causis et signis diuturnorum morborum libri II.*
(f. 38) *De curatione acutorum morborum libri II.*
(f. 61) *De curatione diuturnorum morborum libri II* (Expl. *wie im* Phillipps. 1531) (see p. 17).

Leipzig, Universitätsbibliothek, 64; s. XVIII.
= Cod. graec. 64 (*Census*: 108, nr [0468]).

Apollonius Citiensis: (p. 1) *Commentarius in Hippocratis de articulis, libri III.*

Leipzig, Universitätsbibliothek, 65; s. XIX.
= Cod. graec. 65 (*Census*: 108, nr [0469]).

Aëtius Amidenus: (p. 1) *Iatricorum libri XVI* (L. IX. X).

Leipzig, Universitätsbibliothek, 66; s. XVII.
= Cod. graec. 66 (*Census*: 108, nr [0470]).

Stephanus Alexandrinus: (f. 1 *De sacra divinaque arte auri faciendi* (Περὶ χρυσοποιΐας).
Cleopatra: (f. 112) *De mensuris et ponderibus.*

Lesbos, Βιβλ. τῆς τοῦ Λειμῶνος Μονῆς
Now Καλλονή Λέσβου, Βιβλιοθήκη τῆς τοῦ Λειμῶνος Μονῆς

Lesbos, Βιβλ. τῆς τοῦ Λειμῶνος Μονῆς, 175; s. XVII.
Καλλονή Λέσβου, Βιβλιοθήκη τῆς τοῦ Λειμῶνος Μονῆς, 175.

Epiphanius, **Gregorius Nyssenus**, **Meletius monachus**: *Excerpta varia.*

Lesbos, Βιβλ. τῆς τοῦ Λειμῶνος Μονῆς, 268; a. 1552.
Καλλονή Λέσβου, Βιβλιοθήκη τῆς τοῦ Λειμῶνος Μονῆς, 268.

Asclepiades: (nr 24) *Praecepta salubria.*

Leyden, Universitäts-Bibliothek
Now Leiden, Universiteitsbibliotheek

Leyden, Universitäts-Bibliothek, (Catal. p. 395); s. XV.
= *Vossianus graecus* in quarto 9 (now VGQ 9) (*Census*: 109, nr [0474]).
See also **Voss. 4° 9** below (p. 60).

Rufus:
De medicamentis purgantibus.
De vesicae renumque affectibus.

Leyden, Universitäts-Bibliothek, B. P., 2 A; s. XVI.
= Bibliotheca Publica Graeca 2 A (now BPG 2 A) (*Census*: 109, nr [0475]).

Stephanus Atheniensis: *Enarratio Galeni de methodo medendi ad Glauconem librorum.*

Leyden, Universitäts-Bibliothek, B. P., 6; s. XIV.
= Bibliotheca Publica Graeca 6 (now BPG 6) (*Census*: 109, nr [0476]).

Aëtius Amidenus: *Iatricorum libri XVI* (Libri IV).

Leyden, Universitäts-Bibliothek, B. P., 62 A; s. XV.
= Bibliotheca Publica Graeca 62 (now BPG 62 A) (*Census*: 109, nr [0478]).

Muscio: *De morbis mulierum.*

Leyden, Universitäts-Bibliothek, Gron., 12; s. XVI.
= *Gronovianus* 12 (now GRO 12) (*Census*: 109, nr [0480]).

Gregorius Nyssenus: (f. 244) *De hominis opificio* (Expl. cap. 23 καὶ εἴ τις ἐκ τῆς ἀνάγκης ταύτης ἀΐδ...).

Leyden, Universitäts-Bibliothek, Ruhnken, 11; s. XVIII.
= *Ruhnkenianus* 11 (now RUH 11) (*Census*: 110, nr [0481]).

Meletius monachus: *De natura hominis.*

Leyden, Universitäts-Bibliothek, Vossian.
= *Vossianus graecus* in octavo 19 (now VGO 19) (*Census*: 110, nr [0485]).

Hermes Trismegistus: *De succis plantarum.*

Leyden, Universitäts-Bibliothek, Vossian. 29; s. –.
= *Vossianus graecus* in folio 29 (now VGF 29) (*Census*: 111, nr [0492]).

Aelius Promotus: *Physica et antipathetica.*

Leyden, Universitäts-Bibliothek, Voss. 4° 9; s. XIV, XVI.
= *Vossianus graecus* in quarto 9 (now VGQ 9) (*Census*: 112, nr [0497]).
See also **(Catal. p. 395)** above (p. 59).

Rufus:
De medicamentis purgantibus.
De vesicae renumque affectibus (*Vgl.* Bodleian. Catal. mss. Angl. et Hib. I 1 nr 2182).

Leyden, Universitäts-Bibliothek, Voss. 4° 54; s. XIII.
= *Vossianus graecus* in quarto 54 (now VGQ 54) (*Census*: 113, nr [0502]).

Hypatus: (f. 315–316) *Interpretatio partium corporis.*

Leyden, Universitäts-Bibliothek, Voss. 8° 18; s. XVI.
= *Vossianus graecus* in octavo 18 (now VGO 18) (*Census*: 113, nr [0504]).

Aëtius Amidenus: *Excerpta varia.*
Soranus:
De matrice et muliebri pudendo (*Vgl.* Soranus ed. Ermerins praef. p. CX).
De muliebribus affectionibus.

Leyden, Universitäts-Bibliothek, Voss. 8° 20; s. XV.
= *Vossianus graecus* in octavo 20 (now VGO 20) (*Census*: 113, nr [0505]).

Xenocrates: (f. 1–58) *De morte* (fine mutil.).

Leyden, Universitäts-Bibliothek, Voss. fol. 10; s. XVI.
= *Vossianus graecus* in folio 10 (now VGF 10) (*Census*: 113, nr [0506]).

Soranus: *Hippocratis genus et vita secundum Soranum* (*Vgl.* Hipp. Ed. Ermerins prf. p. IX).

Leyden, Universitäts-Bibliothek, Voss. fol. 22; s. XV.
= *Vossianus graecus* in folio 22 (now VGF 22) (*Census*: 114, nr [0508]).

Paulus Aegineta: *Epitomae medicae libri septem* (Libri V).

Leyden, Universitäts-Bibliothek, Voss. fol. 25; s. XV.
= *Vossianus graecus* in folio 25 (now VGF 25) (*Census*: 114, nr [0509]).

Democritus: *De sympathicis et antipathicis.*
Heliodorus: *De mensuris et ponderibus.*

Leyden, Universitäts-Bibliothek, Voss. fol. 31; s. XV.
= *Vossianus graecus* in folio 31 (now VGF 31) (*Census*: 114, nr [0511]).

Theophilus: *De pulsibus* (Frgm. Inc. Ἐπὶ τῶν πυρεκτικῶν σωμάτων).

Leyden, Universitäts-Bibliothek, Voss. fol. 32; s. –.
= *Vossianus graecus* in folio 32 (now VGF 32) (*Census*: 114, nr [0512]).

Ioannes Zacharias Actuarius:
De spiritu animali libri II.

De urinis libri VII.
De methodo medendi Libri VI (L. I–V).

Leyden, Universitäts-Bibliothek, Voss. fol. 58; s. XV.
= *Vossianus graecus* in folio 58 (now VGF 58) (*Census*: 114, nr [0514]).

Aëtius Amidenus: *Iatricorum libri XVI* (Frgm. ex l. I. III. IV. V. VII. VIII).
Dioscurides: *De materia medica* (Lib. I).

Leyden, Universitäts-Bibliothek, Voss. fol. 59; s. XIV.
= *Vossianus graecus* in folio 59 (now VGF 59) (*Census*: 114, nr [0515]).

Dioscurides:
Liber agens de experientia medica, de simplicibus et compositis medicamentis, ordine literarum digestus.
Excerpta (De divisione partium anni et quaenam medicinae singulis conveniant temporibus sec. Aegyptios).
Metaphrasis in Nicandri Theriaca et Alexipharmaca.
Theophilus: *De pulsibus.*

Leyden, Universitäts-Bibliothek, Vossian. fol. 65; s. XV.
= *Vossianus graecus* in folio 65 (now VGF 65) (*Census*: 114, nr [0516]).

Synesius: *De febribus.*

Leyden, Universitäts-Bibliothek, Voss. misc. 22.
= *Vossianus miscellaneus* 22 (now VMI 22) (*Census*: 115, nr [0519]).

Xenocrates: *De alimento ex aquatilibus.*

London, British Museum
Now London, British Library

London, British Museum, Addit. 5108; s. XV ex.

Diodorus: (f. 4^{v}) *De mensuris et ponderibus.*

London, British Museum, Addit. 8231; s. XVII.

Dioscurides: (f. 1) *Excerpta* (Frgm. Ὀνομαστικὸν εἰς τὰ τοῦ Δ. π. ὕ. ἰ. Inc. Αἰβαδανέ. Expl. ὤκιμον).

London, British Museum, Addit. 10, 058; s. XV.

Soranus: (f. 46) *De ponderibus et mensuris* (Inc. Τῶν μέτρων καὶ σταθμῶν οὐ μόνον. Expl. ὁ ξέστης ⱶ' ἆς":).
Lucas: (f. 46ᵛ) *Compositio salsi intinctus.*
Gregorius Theologus: (f. 47) *Alatium.*
Aëtius Amidenus: (f. 101ᵛ) *Excerpta varia.*
Paulus Aegineta:
(f. 102) *Excerpta varia* (Exc. apud Anonymum π. δυνάμεως ζουλαπίων καὶ ἑτέρων πομάτων).
(f. 151) *De succedaneis, ex Galeno* (Expl. ὤκιμον τὸ βασιλικόν).
Andromachus: (f. 161ᵛ) *Theriaca* (manu recentiore).

London, British Museum, Londin. Addit. (Brit. Mus.) 14620; s. IX.

Epiphanius: *De mensuris et ponderibus II.*

London, British Museum, Londin. Addit. (Brit. Mus.) 17148; s. VII.

Epiphanius: *De mensuris et ponderibus II.*

London, British Museum, Addit. 17, 900; s. XVII.

Alexander Rex: (f. 89ᵛ) *De septem herbarum facultate.*
Theophilus:
(f. 95) *De urinis.*
(f. 101ᵛ) *De alvi excrementis.*
Dioscurides: (f. 268ᵛ) *Liber agens de experientia medica, de simplicibus et compositis medicamentis, ordine literarum digestus.*
Ioannes Episcopus Prisdianensis: (f. 271) *Collectanea de excrementis.*

London, British Museum, Arundel. 537; s. XV in.

Ioannes Zacharias Actuarius:
(f. 1) *De urinis libri VII* (Inc. ποικίλης = Idel. II 4, 10).
(f. 156) *De spiritu animali libri II.*
(f. 196ᵛ) *De methodo medendi libri VI* (Expl. ἀποσιτίαι καὶ ἄλγη = Id. II 405, 28).

London, British Museum, Burneian. 75; s. XV.

Marcellus Sidetes: (f. 164ᵛ) *Medicina ex piscibus.*

London, British Museum, Burneian. 94; s. XV–XVI, XV (XVI).

Lycus: *Excerpta varia* (Ὅτι οὐκ ἐφικνεῖται τὸ σύμμετρον αἰδοῖον τοῦ ἄρρενος τοῦ στομίου τῆς ὑστέρας. Inc. Τοῦ κύτους τῆς μήτρας. Expl. βολῆς τινος προσδεῖν. *Aus* Oribas. III 382).

Rufus:

(f. 154) *De corporis humani appellationibus* (*Vollständig*).

(f. 161ᵛ) *Nomenclatura rerum ad hominem pertinentium. Libri III.*

Oribasius: (f. 170) *Medicae collectiones ad Iulianum* (L. XXIV. XXV. Expl. ἀλλὰ καὶ βολῆς τινος προσδεῖν).

Rufus: (f. 197ᵛ) *De corporis humani appellationibus* (*Excerpte.* Inc. Ἀναγκαιότατόν ἐστι προδιδαχθῆναι. Expl. ἀνάλογον τοῖς ἐν χερσίν · οὕτω δὲ καὶ ὅσα).

London, British Museum, Harleian. 5626; s. XV (XVI), XV (XVI ?), XV–XVI, XV–XVI (?).

Aëtius Amidenus: (f. 1) *Iatricorum libri XVI* (L. III).

Adamantius: (f. 2) *Excerpta varia.*

Antyllus, Archigenes, Iustus, Logadius, Rufus: (f. 2) *Excerpta varia* (Ἰατροσόφιον ποιηθὲν ὑπὸ διαφόρων φιλοσόφων τῶν πρὸς Ἱπποκράτους γιγνομένων αὐτοῦ μαθητῶν Ἀντίλλου, Ἀρχιγένους, Ἰούστου, Λογαδίου, Ῥούφου).

London, British Museum, Harleian. 5679; s. XV.

Dioscurides:

(f. 2) *De materia medica* (Libri II titul. et prooem. desunt).

(f. 209) *De venenis eorumque praecautione et medicatione* (in tit. om. καὶ θεραπείας).

London, British Museum, Harleian. 5685; s. XII–XI (s. XIII *nach M. Thompson*).

Nemesius Emesenus: (f. 1) *De natura hominis.*

London, British Museum, Harleian. 6295; s. XV (XIV sec. catal.), XV (XIV).

Alexander Aphrodisiensis: *Problematum physicorum et medicorum eclogae. Libri V*:

(f. 1) Expl. ἐνδιδόναι τῆς οἰκείας ὁρμῆς καὶ φορᾶς.

(f. 25) L. IV et V.

Gregorius Nyssenus: (f. 88ᵛ) *De pulsibus.*

Mercurius monachus: (f. 111ᵛ) *De pulsibus.*

London, British Museum, Harleian. 6305; s. XVI, XVI (?).

Aëtius Amidenus: (f. 3 [?]) *Excerpta varia* (Inc. Ἐγὼ δὲ διὰ παντὸς τῷ διὰ τῶν κωδίων χρῶμαι).
Paulus Aegineta: (f. 151 [?]) *De succedaneis, ex Galeno.*
Dioscurides: (f. 157^{v}) *De mensuris et ponderibus.*
Paulus Aegineta: (f. 159) *De mensuris et ponderibus* (Expl. διαφορά = Ald. f. 138^{v}, 18).
Theophilus: (f. 161) *Excerpta varia* (Θεραπεία μελαινῶν ἀλφῶν. Inc. Ὁ δὲ ἐν Ἀσίᾳ ὑπό τινος ἀγοραίου. Expl. πινόμενος μετὰ οἴνου ἀτοκίαν καὶ αὐτό ποιεῖ).

London, British Museum, Harleian. 6326; s. XVI ex.

Aretaeus:
(f. 2) *De causis et signis acutorum morborum libri II.*
(f. 48^{v}) *De causis et signis diuturnorum morborum libri II.*
(f. 18) *De curatione acutorum morborum libri II.*
(f. 183^{v}) *De causis et signis diuturnorum morborum libri II* (Lib. I usque ad c. 13 γάλακτι).

London, British Museum, Regius 16. C. XVI; s. XVI.
Now Royal. 16.C.xvi (*Census*: 120, nr [0556]).

Artemidorus: (f. 8) *De urinis* (»mit lat. Interlinearübersetzung.« Kalbfleisch).

London, British Museum, Sloan. 804; s. XVI (?).

Dioscurides: (f. 2) *De facile parabilibus tam simplicibus quam compositis medicamentis libri II.*

London, British Museum, Sloan. 2434; s. XVII (?).

Aëtius Amidenus: (f. 1. 19^{v}. 51. 104) *Iatricorum libri XVI* (Frgm.).

London, Medical Society
Now at the Wellcome Library, London

London, Medical Society, A Ac 2 = Wf 15; s. XV in.
Now London, Wellcome Library, MS. MSL 114 (*Census*: 121, nr [0563]).

Paulus Aegineta: *Epitomae medicae libri septem* (L. I–VII. Expl. ψὼς ὅ ἐστι κόρος, μο^{δι} λ̄).

London, Medical Society, HHi 17 = We 30; s. XV in.
Now London, Wellcome Library, MS. MSL 60 (*Census*: 121, nr [0564]).

Ioannes Zacharias Actuarius: *De urinis libri VII* (Frgm. ex l. I. VI. VII).
Paulus Aegineta:
(f. 50) *De succedaneis, ex Galeno* (Expl. ἀντὶ ᾠοῦ τὸ λευκὸν γάλα γυναικίῳ).
(nr 21 Dbg.) *Excerpta varia* (Remedia).
Stephanus Atheniensis: (nr 24 Dbg.) *De febrium differentiis ex ore Theophili* (Expl. *wie im* Berol. Phillipps. [1532] [see p. 18]). »Est opus traditum sub nomine Palladii«).
Theophilus:
(nr 28 Dg.) *De urinis*.
(nr 39 Dbg.) *De pulsibus* (Expl. τὰ δὲ ἄλλα φυλάττουσι κατὰ φύσιν).

London, Medical Society, HH i 21. 22 = We 28. 29; s. XV.
Now London, Wellcome Library, MS. MSL 52 A&B (*Census*: 121, nr [0565]).

Ioannes Zacharias Actuarius:
(f. 1) *De spiritu animali libri II*.
(f. 44) *De urinis libri VII*.
(f. 145–257[v]) *De methodo medendi Libri VI*.
Aëtius Amidenus: (f. 346) *Excerpta varia* (*Wie im* cod. Gallipoli 38. Expl. τάσιν τινὰ τῆς ἀρτηρίας βραχεῖαν).
Theophilus: (f. 354[v]) *De alvi excrementis*.

London, Medical Society, H Hi 23 = We 32a; s. XV in.
Now London, Wellcome Library, MS. MSL 62 (*Census*: 121, nr [0566]).

Aretaeus:
De causis et signis acutorum morborum libri II.
De curatione acutorum morborum libri II.
De causis et signis diuturnorum morborum libri II.
De curatione acutorum morborum libri II.
De curatione diuturnorum morborum libri II (L. II c. 2. 23. 5–7).
Rufus:
(nr 2 Dbg., Not. et Extr.) *De corporis humani appellationibus* (Expl. ἐνδεχόμενον, καὶ ἡ τῶν ὀστέων φύσις).
(nr 2 Dbg., Not. et Extr.) *Nomenclatura rerum ad hominem pertinentium. Libri III*.

London, Medical Society, NNa 11 = Wf 8; s. –.
Now London, Wellcome Library, MS. MSL 112 (*Census*: 121, nr [0567]).

Ioannes Zacharias Actuarius: *De methodo medendi libri VI* (Inc. Ἡ μὲν παροιμία φησί, χελώνης. Expl. ἐνταῦθά πη συγκαταπαύειν).

London, Medical Society, We 29; s. XV ex.
Now London, Wellcome Library, MS. MSL 52 B (*Census*: 121, nr [0568]).

Herodotus: (f. 366–403) *Diagnostica de morbis acutis et chronicis* (Expl. καὶ εἰ μὲν παρηγοροῖντο, ἐάσομεν · εἰ δὲ παροξύνοιντο = Parisin. Suppl. 636 [above p. 140]. f. 61ᵛ, 15).

London, Medical Society, Wf 6; s. –.
Now London, Wellcome Library, MS. MSL 126 (*Census*: 121, nr [0569]).

Oribasius: *Medicae collectiones ad Iulianum* (L. I–X. XIV).

London, Medical Society, Wf 7; s. XVI.
Now London, Wellcome Library, MS. MSL 109 (*Census*: 121, nr [0570]).

Aëtius Amidenus: *Iatricorum libri XVI* (L. IX–XV).

London, Medical Society, Wf 16; s. XVI ex.
Now London, Wellcome Library, MS. MSL 124 (*Census*: 122, nr [0571]).

Ioannes Zacharias Actuarius: *De urinis libri VII.*

Lyon

Lyon, Bibliothèque de la ville, 52; s. XVI–XVII.
Now Bibliothèque municipale, 122 (*Census*: 123, nr [0572]).

Nemesius Emesenus: (f. 134) *De natura hominis* (Frgm. Theodoreti, Cyri episcopi, Nemesii etc. excerpta et interrogationes de rebus theologicis).

Madrid

Madrid, Matrit. 166.
= Madrid, Biblioteca Nacional, Vitr. 26–1 (*Census*: 124, nr [0573]).
See also **9715** and **N 116 (olim Toletanus 97.15)** below (p. 70).

Ioannes Damascenus: (f. 212) *Excerpta* («Ex Isaaci libro videntur desumpta» Wellmann).

Madrid, Bibl. Univ.
Now Madrid, Biblioteca de la Universidad Complutense

Madrid, Bibl. Univ., 30; s. XI.
Now Biblioteca de la Universidad Complutense, 116-zo-22 (*Census*: 124, nr [0574]).

Epiphanius: (nr III) *De mensuris et ponderibus.*

Madrid, Nationalbibliothek
Madrid, Biblioteca Nacional

Madrid, Nationalbibliothek, 4581 (olim N 45); s. XII.
= 4581 (*Census*: 125, nr [0576]).

Paulus Aegineta: *Epitomae medicae libri septem*:
(f. 1) L. IV inde a cap. 56.
(f. 3^{v}. 28^{v}. 124) L. V. VI. VII.

Madrid, Nationalbibliothek, 4616 (olim N 48); s. XV.
= 4616 (*Census*: 125, nr [0577]).
See also **4616 (olim N 84)** below.

Petosiris: (f. 89. 90) *Epistula ad regem Nechepso.*

Madrid, Nationalbibliothek, 4616 (olim N 84); s. XV.
Same as **4616 (olim N 48)** above.
= 4616 (*Census*: 125, nr [0578]).

Alexander Aphrodisiensis: (f. 46^{v}, 54^{v}) *Problematum physicorum et medicorum eclogae. Libri V.*

Cassius iatrosophistes: (f. 55) *Quaestiones medicae et problemata physica* (Frgm. ex Cassii probl. XII. XX. XXIII. XXXV. LXIII. LXIV).
Pythagoras: (f. 66, 74ᵛ, 80ᵛ, 82ᵛ, 83ᵛ, 84ᵛ, 86ᵛ, 87, 87ᵛ) *Supputationes prognosticae.*
Petosiris: (f. 89. 90) *Epistula ad regem Nechepso.*
Dioscurides: (f. 171) *Excerpta* (Περί τινων βοτανῶν δυνάμεως. Inc. Ἀψίνθιον θερμόν ἐστι).
Paulus Aegineta:
(f. 132) *Excerpta varia.*
(f. 132) *Epitomae medicae libri septem* (Frgm. Liber VII c. 1–3).

Madrid, Nationalbibliothek, 4631 (N 110); a. 1474.
= 4631 (*Census*: 125, nr [0579]).

Hermes Trismegistus: (f. 6) *Kyranides.*
Harpocration:
(f. 6ᵛ. 37. 53ᵛ. 67) *De facultatibus naturalibus animalium et herbarum et lapidum* (A–Y. »Consutum cum Hermetis Trismegisti Κυρανίδες.« Wellmann).
(f. 75) *Epistula ad imperatorem.*
Paulus Aegineta:
(f. 86) *Epitomae medicae libri septem* (Liber VII c. 1–3 »alienis additis«. Wellmann).
(f. 86) *Excerpta varia.*
Dioscurides: (f. 89) *Excerpta* (Περὶ δυνάμεώς τινων βοτανῶν κατ᾽ ἀλφ. Inc. Ἀλθαία ἢν ἔνιοι).
Paulus Aegineta: (f. 147ᵛ) *De succedaneis, ex Galeno.*
Epiphanius: (f. 153) *De duodecim gemmis panno sacerdotis infibulatis.*
Dioscurides: (f. 155) *Excerpta* (Περὶ λίθων).
Aëtius Amidenus: (f. 155) *Excerpta varia* (Inscr. Π. λίθων Διοσκορίδου. impress. Iriarte).
Pythagoras: (f. 158. 159ᵛ) *Supputationes prognosticae.*

Madrid, Nationalbibliothek, 4636; s. XV.
See also **4636 (ol. N 115)** below.

Hypatus: (f. 209) *Interpretatio partium corporis* (Sine auctoris nomine. Inscr. Περὶ τῶν μελῶν τοῦ ἀνθρωπίνου σώματος. Inc. *wie im* Scorial. [Σ. I. 12] [above p. 34]).

Madrid, Nationalbibliothek, 4636 (ol. N 115); s. XV.
Same as **4636** above.
= 4636 (*Census*: 125, nr [0582]).

Rufus: (f. 209) *De corporis humani appellationibus* (Frgm.).

Madrid, Nationalbibliothek, 4759 (olim N 138); s. XVI.
= 4759 (*Census*: 126, nr [0583]).

Diocles: (f. 137) *Ad Antigonum regem epistula de tuenda valetitudine.*
Nemesius Emesenus: (f. 167) *De natura hominis.*

Madrid, Nationalbibliothek, 4861; s. XVI.

Gregorius Nyssenus: (no. VI) *De hominis opificio* (Π. εἰκόν. ἀνθρ.).

Madrid, Nationalbibliothek, 9715; s. –.
= Vitr. 26–1 (*Census*: 126, nr [0586]).
See also **Matrit. 166** above (p. 68) and **N 116 (olim Toletanus 97.15)** below.

Ioannes Zacharias Actuarius: *Tractatus de urinis, qui ex Avicenna translatus dicitur in graecam linguam a Christodulo, in ordinem redactus ab Actuario Zacharia.*

Madrid, Nationalbibliothek, N 116 (olim Toletanus 97.15); s. XV.
= Vitr. 26–1 (*Census*: 126–127, nr [0587]).
Same as **Matrit. 166** (p. 68) and **9715** above.

Philo: (f. 214v) *Excerpta varia* (Ἀντίδοτος ἡ τοῦ Φίλωνος).

Madrid, Bibliothek des Königs

Madrid, Privatbibliothek des Königs, 14 (olim 13); s. XVI.
Now Salamanca, Biblioteca universitaria, 2710 (*Census*: 127, nr [0588]).

Gregorius Nyssenus: (f. 1) *De hominis opificio* (*Wie im* cod. [Madrid] Bibl. Nac. [4861]) (see p. 70).

Madrid, Privatbibliothek des Königs, 44 (olim 23); s. XV ex.
Now Salamanca, Biblioteca universitaria, 2659 (*Census*: 127, nr [0589]).

Dioscurides:
(f. 13) *De materia medica.*

(f. 164ᵛ) *De venenis eorumque praecautione et medicatione.*
(f. 171) *De iis, quae virus eiaculantur, animalibus libellus, in quo et de rabioso cane.*

Galenos: (f. 180ᵛ) *De theriaca* (π. τῆς μεγάλης θηριακῆς τῆς δι' ἐχιδνῶν. Inc. Πολλῆς οὔσης διαφωνίας περὶ τὰς γραφικὰς ἀποδείξεις. Expl. δεῖ δὲ σαρκῶν μὲν δύο μέρη βάλλεσθαι, ἄρτων δὲ ἕν).

Mailand, Archivio del Capitolo Metropolitano
Milano, Archivio del Capitolo Metropolitano

Mailand, Arch. del Capitolo Metropolitano, 2; s. XV.
= Milano, Archivio del Capitolo Metropolitano, II, E 2, 17 (*Census*: 128, nr [0590]).

Synesius: (f. 2) *Epistula de silphio ad fratrem.*
Dioscurides:
(f. 11–113ᵛ) *De materia medica.*
(f. 114–119) *De venenis eorumque praecautione et medicatione* (in tit. om. καὶ θεραπείας; *vgl. den* [Lond.] Harleian. [5679] [p. 64]).
(f. 119ᵛ–126) *De iis, quae virus eiaculantur, animalibus libellus, in quo et de rabioso cane.*
Neophytus Prodromenus: (f. 129–132ᵛ) *Remediorum collectio alphabetica* (Expl. ὤκυμον τὸ βασιλικόν).
Paulus Aegineta: (f. 135ᵛ–137) *De succedaneis, ex Galeno.*
Dioscurides:
(f. 137ᵛ–139) *De mensuris et ponderibus* (Expl. σταθμοῦ δὲ ὁλκαὶ ρκ').
(f. 139–143ᵛ) *Excerpta* (»Un indice dei nomi delle piante di D. coi relative num. distribuite, almeno in parte, secondo i luoghi nei quali nascono«).

Mailand, Bibl. Ambrosiana
Milano, Biblioteca Ambrosiana

Mailand, Bibl. Ambrosiana (*bei* Berthelot Ruelle, p. 56).
= ? **E 37 Sup.** (p. 74), **A 57 inf.** (p. 78), or **A 193 Inf.** (p. 79) (*Census*: 128, nr [0592]).

Synesius: *Ad Dioscorum, scholia in librum Democriti.*

Mailand, Bibl. Ambrosiana, Ambros. duo (*Vgl.* Montfaucon I p. 504).
= ? **H 22 sup.** (p. 75) and **& 141 Sup.** (p. 78). respectively) (*Census*: 128–129, nr [0594]).

Rufus: *De corporis humani appellationibus.*

Mailand, Bibl. Ambrosiana, A 45 Sup.; s. XIII.

Pythagoras: (f. 45ᵛ) *Prognostica.*

Mailand, Bibl. Ambrosiana, A 92 Sup.; s. XV–XVI.

Cassius iatrosophistes: (f. 45) *Quaestiones medicae et problemata physica.*

Mailand, Bibl. Ambrosiana, A 95 Sup.; s. XV.

Dioscurides:
(f. 18) *De mensuris et ponderibus.*
(f. 19–49ᵛ) *De materia medica* (alph.).
Theophilus: (f. 52) *De urinis* (= Idel. I 261–264, 20).
Dioscurides:
(f. 92–95) *De materia medica* (alph.).
(f. 104–150) *De materia medica* (alph.).
(f. 129ᵛ–133ᵛ) *De venenis eorumque praecautione et medicatione.*
Theophilus: (f. 165) *Commentarius in Hippocratis aphorismos* (= »Dietz II 245 sub finem, 247, 7–300,15 passim«).

Mailand, Bibl. Ambrosiana, A 157 Sup.; s. X (XI ?).
= A 175 Sup (nicht A 157).

Aëtius Amidenus: *Excerpta varia.*

Mailand, Bibl. Ambrosiana, A 162 Sup.; s. XV.

Aglaias: (f. 69) *Ad suffusiones Aglaiae ..., Alexandri discipuli, condicipuli Demosthenis et amici, versus heroelegi* (Expl. σύνθεσις ἥδε πέλει).

Mailand, Bibl. Ambrosiana, A 175 Sup.
See also **A 157 Sup**. above.

Aëtius Amidenus: *Excerpta varia.*

Mailand, Bibl. Ambrosiana, B 39 Sup.; s. XIV–XV.

Nemesius Emesenus: (f. 26) *De natura hominis* (Frgm.).

Mailand, Bibl. Ambrosiana, B 63 Sup.; s. XIV ex.

Gregorius Nyssenus: (f. 87) *De hominis opificio* (Sine auct. nomine. Expl. c. 30 ἔστι δὲ καὶ ἄλλα τινά = Migne p. 241 A).

Mailand, Bibl. Ambrosiana, B 72 Sup.; s. –.
s. XV.

Synesius: (f. 1 ff.) *Epistula de silphio ad fratrem.*

Mailand, Bibl. Ambrosiana, B 82 Sup.; s. XVI.

Gregorius Nyssenus: (f. 1) *De hominis opificio* (Expl. c. 22 τὴν τοῦ ἀδὰμ κλῆσιν).

Mailand, Bibl. Ambrosiana, B 113 Sup.; s. XIV in.

Theophilus: (f. 4) *Commentarius in Hippocratis aphorismos* (= Dietz II 245–543).
Palladius: (f. 85) *Scholia in Hippocratis de popularibus morbis librum sextum, sectiones VIII.*
Paulus Aegineta: (f. 229ᵛ) *Excerpta varia* (Π. δυνάμεως τοῦ πηγάνου. Inc. Πηγάνου ἐν ταῖς βοτάναις πάσαις).

Mailand, Bibl. Ambrosiana, B 126 Sup.; s. XIV, XIV ex.

Paulus Aegineta: *Epitomae medicae libri septem*:
(f. 1) L. I–VII 2.
(f. 143) L. III 21.

Mailand, Bibl. Ambrosiana, B 157 Sup.; s. XV–XVI.

Aretaeus:
(f. 1) *De causis et signis acutorum morborum libri II* (Inc. a l. I c. 6).
(f. 24ᵛ) *De causis et signis diuturnorum morborum libri II.*
(f. 70) *De curatione acutorum morborum libri II.*
(f. 111ᵛ) *De curatione diuturnorum morborum libri II* (non pauca desunt).

Mailand, Bibl. Ambrosiana, C 69 Sup.; s. XV, XVI.

Cyrillus Alexandrinus: (f. 34) *De mensuris et ponderibus* (Περὶ μετρικῶν ὀνομάτων [Treu]).

Mailand, Bibl. Ambrosiana, C 88 Sup.; s. X in.

Gregorius Nyssenus: (f. 54) *De hominis opificio* (Expl. ἐπιτεχνηθέντος τῇ ὕλῃ = Migne p. 253 C).

Mailand, Bibl. Ambrosiana, C 89 Sup.; s. –.

Ioannes Zacharias Actuarius: (f. 1) *De urinis libri VII* (»Deest magna pars libri I«).

Mailand, Bibl. Ambrosiana, C 102 Sup.; s. XV.

Dioscurides: (f. 1–29) *De materia medica* (Περὶ ἐπιστήμης ἰατρικῆς τὸ περὶ βοτάνων βιβλίον α'. Expl. τὰ πρὸς ὀξυδορκίαν ὀφθαλμικά).

Mailand, Bibl. Ambrosiana, C 119 Sup.; s. XV.
= *L 119 sup. and not C 119 sup.*
Same as **L 119 Sup** below (p. 76).

Dioscurides: *De materia medica* (Libri VII).

Mailand, Bibl. Ambrosiana, D 13 Sup.; s. –.

Oribasius: (f. 1) *Conspectus ad Eustathium filium. Libri II.*
Ioannes Episcopus Prisdianensis: (f. 300^v) *Collectanea de urinis* (Inscr. man. rec. Ὀριβασίου π. οὔρων, in mg. Ἰωάννου ἐπισκόπου Πρισδριανῶν. Inc. Ἡ θεία φύσις ποιήσασα τὸν ἄνθρωπον. Expl. mutil.: ἐν τῷ οὔρῳ φαινόμενα τῆς κύστεως...).
Oribasius: (f. 300^v) *Excerpta varia* (Περὶ οὔρων. Inc. Ἡ θεία φύσις ποιήσασα τὸν ἄνθρωπον. Expl. mutil. ἐν τῷ οὔρῳ φαινόμενα, τῆς κύστεως ... Inscr. man. rec. Ὀριβασίου περὶ οὔρων, in mg. ῥ Ἰωάννου ἐπισκόπου Πρισδριανῶν).

Mailand, Bibl. Ambrosiana, D 33 Sup.; s. XV.

Mercurius monachus: (f. 66) *De pulsibus* (Expl. μίαν καὶ δύο = Ideler p. 255, 27).

Mailand, Bibl. Ambrosiana, E 37 Sup.; s. XVI.
See also **(*bei* Berthelot Ruelle, p. 56)** above (p. 71).

Zosimus Panopolita: (f. 290^v) *Liber de virtute et compositione aquarum.*
Synesius: (f. 301) *Ad Dioscorem.*
Stephanus Alexandrinus: (f. 308^v) *De sacra divinaque arte auri faciendi.*
Alexander Rex: (f. 351) *De septem herbarum facultate.*

Mailand, Bibl. Ambrosiana, F 88 Sup.; s. XV.

Nemesius Emesenus: (f. 163^v) *De natura hominis* (Expl. δόγμασι παραλειπτέον = 144, 10 Matth.).

Mailand, Bibl. Ambrosiana, F 107 Sup.; s. X.

Gregorius Nyssenus: (f. 75) *De hominis opificio* (Frgm.).

Mailand, Bibl. Ambrosiana, G 69 Sup.; s. XV.

Oribasius: (f. 341) *Excerpta varia*.

Mailand, Bibl. Ambrosiana, H 11 Sup.; s. XIII.

Gregorius Nyssenus: (f. 265) *De hominis opificio*.

Mailand, Bibl. Ambrosiana, H 22 Sup.; s. XV.
See also **Ambros. duo (*Vgl.* Montfaucon I p. 504)** above (p. 71).

Rufus: (f. 11 *und* 12ᵛ) *De corporis humani appellationibus.*

Mailand, Bibl. Ambrosiana, H 43 Sup.; s. XV–XVI.

Alexander Aphrodisiensis: (f. 110) *Quarundam difficultatum solutiones.*

Mailand, Bibl. Ambrosiana, H 49 Sup.; s. –.

Diocles: (f. 16) *Ad Antigonum regem epistula de tuenda valetitudine.*

Mailand, Bibl. Ambrosiana, L 30 Sup.; a. 1524.

Theophilus: (f. 1) *Commentarius in Hippocratis aphorismos* (= Dietz II 245–543, 4. »Falso Philotheus pro Theophilo scriptum est«).
Stephanus Alexandrinus: (f. 127) *Scholia in Hippocratis praenotiones. Sectiones III.*

Mailand, Bibl. Ambrosiana, L 44 Sup.; s. XIV ex.

Synesius: (f. 1ff.) *Epistula de silphio ad fratrem*.

Mailand, Bibl. Ambrosiana, L 110 Sup.; s. XVI.

Theophilus:
(f. 1) *Commentarius in Hippocratis aphorismos* (»In prooemio non semper verba eadem atque apud Dietz II 245.
(f. 117) *De urinis* (»Falso Philotheus pro Theophilo scriptum est«).
Stephanus Atheniensis: (f. 131) *Enarratio Galeni de methodo medendi ad Glauconem librorum* (Inc. Τὸ προοίμιον δύο ταῦτα ...).

Theophilus: (f. 173) *De hominis fabrica libri V* (Expl. mutil. τὸν ἀδένα ἔχοντες, τὸ δὲ σχῆμα. *Vgl. den* [Berol.] Phillipps. [1527] [above p. 17]).
Soranus: (f. 233) *Hippocratis genus et vita secundum Soranum.*

Mailand, Bibl. Ambrosiana, L 119 Sup.; s. XV.
See also **C 119 Sup.** above (p. 74).

Dioscurides:
De materia medica (not C 119 Sup.).
(f. 177^{v}) *De venenis eorumque praecautione et medicatione.*
(f. 186) *De iis, quae virus eiaculantur, animalibus libellus, in quo et de rabioso cane.*

Mailand, Bibl. Ambrosiana, M 41 sup.; s. XV.

Alexander Aphrodisiensis: (f. 130) *Problematum physicorum et medicorum eclogae. Libri V.*

Mailand, Bibl. Ambrosiana, O 117 Sup.; s. –.
s. XV–XVI.

Esdras Propheta: (91^{v}) *De diebus criticis* (Inscr. Περὶ τῶν ἡμερῶν τῶν πεφωτισμένων καὶ ἀφωτίστων. Inc. Εἰσὶν αἱ ἡμέραι, ἃς ἐφανέρωσεν. Expl. ἃς δεῖ παρατηρεῖν).

Mailand, Bibl. Ambrosiana, O 123 Sup.; s. XVI.

Ioannes Zacharias Actuarius: (f. 1) *De methodo medendi libri VI.*

Mailand, Bibl. Ambrosiana, P. 32 Sup.; a. 1564.

Nemesius Emesenus: (f. 1) *De natura hominis* (sub nomine Pachomii).

Mailand, Bibl. Ambrosiana, P 90 Sup.; s. XV–XVI.

Meletius monachus: (f. 4) *De natura hominis.*

Mailand, Bibl. Ambrosiana, Q 13 Sup.; s. –.
s. XV–XVI.

Dioscurides: (f. 285^{v}) *Excerpta varia.*

Mailand, Bibl. Ambrosiana, Q 14 Sup.; s. XV.

Gregorius Nyssenus: (f. 97^{v} [91^{v}]) *De hominis opificio.*

Mailand, Bibl. Ambrosiana, Q 87 Sup.; s. –.
s. XIV–XV, XV.

Dioscurides: (f. 247ᵛ) *Excerpta varia.*
Paulus Aegineta: (f. 271–278ᵛ) *Excerpta varia* (Inc. mutil. ...|ραγία γένηται, μοθοῖς. Expl. γυμνωθῆναι · εἰ μὲν αἱμορ|...).

Mailand, Bibl. Ambrosiana, Q 94 Sup.; s. –.
s. XV–XVI.

Stephanus Atheniensis: (f. 24ᵛ) *De febrium differentiis ex ore Theophili.*
Rufus: (f. 347) *Excerpta varia* (Inc. Κολοκυνθίδος ἐντεριώνης. Expl. εἶτα καὶ τὴν ἀντίδοτον).
Beniaminus: (f. 349–363) *Excerpta.*
Chrysostomius (?): (f. 364ᵛ) *De corporis humani constitutione demonstratio* (»In margine χρυσο$^{c\mu\iota}$.«).
Gregorius Nyssenus: (f. 366ᵛ) *Oratio adversus astronomos* (Wie im [Berol.] Phillipps. [1527] [above p. 17]).

Mailand, Bibl. Ambrosiana, R 20 Sup.; s. –.
s. XV.

Ioannes Zacharias Actuarius:
De spiritu animali libri II.
De urinis libri VII.
De animalibus nocentibus (»enthält die Schrift nicht«. Treu. Also zu streichen).
(f. 20) *De methodo medendi libri VI* (L. I–V).
Mercurius monachus: (f. 533) *De pulsibus.*
Paulus Aegineta: (f. 536) *De succedaneis, ex Galeno.*

Mailand, Bibl. Ambrosiana, R 111 b; s. –.
= **R 111 Sup.** below (*Census*: 133, nr [0654]).

Nepualius: *De sympathicis et antipathicis.*

Mailand, Bibl. Ambrosiana, R 111 Sup.; s. XVI.
See also **R 111 b** above.

Alexander Trallianus: (f. 264) *Epistula de lumbricis.*
Nepualius: (f. 266ᵛ) *De sympathicis et antipathicis.*
Democritus: (f. 268) *De sympathicis et antipathicis.*

Mailand, Bibl. Ambrosiana, S 3 Sup.; s. –, XV ex–XVI in, XVI.
s. XV/XVI, XV-XVI.

Heliodorus: (f. 21) *De mensuris et ponderibus.*
Aelius Promotus:
(f. 21) *Iatrica* (Inc. Ἄλλο βαπτικὸν κικίδια; »Apogr. des Vatic. [graec. 299] [below p. 157]« M. W.; *vgl.* f. 125ᵛ).
(f. 69–112ᵛ) *De animalibus virus eiculantibus et de venenis* (»Stammt aus Vatic. [graec.] 299.« M. W.).
(f. 114) *Physica et antipathetica.*
Nepualius: (f. 117 – 120 b) *De sympathicis et antipathicis.*
Democritus: (f. 122) *De sympathicis et antipathicis* (R 3 Sup. errore Gemoll).
Alexander Trallianus: (f. 170) *Epistula de lumbricis.*

Mailand, Bibl. Ambrosiana, S 19 Sup.; s. –.

Stephanus Atheniensis, Theophilus: *In aphorismos Hippocratis commentarius/ Commentarius in Hippocratis aphorismos* (»Stephani et Theoph. in aphor. Hipp. comm.«).

Mailand, Bibl. Ambrosiana, T 141, s. XVI.
= **& 141 Sup.** below (*Census*: 134, nr [0659]).

Rufus: *De corporis humani appellationibus* (*Vgl.* Daremberg, Ruf. XXIII).

Mailand, Bibl. Ambrosiana, & 141 Sup.; s. XVI.
See also **Ambros. duo (*Vgl.* Montfaucon I p. 504)** (p. 71) and **T 141** above.

Rufus: (f. 1) *De corporis humani appellationibus.*

Mailand, Bibl. Ambrosiana, & 147 Sup.; s. XVI.

Ioannes Zacharias Actuarius: (f. 5ᵛ) *De methodo medendi libri VI* (Inscr. Βιβλίον ἰατρικὸν περιέχον πᾶσαν τέχνην ἐν ἐπιτόμῳ).

Mailand, Bibl. Ambrosiana, A 27 Inf.; s. XVI.

Stephanus Alexandrinus: (f. 2) *Scholia in Hippocratis praenotiones. Sectiones III* (»Operi sine auctoris nomine tradito praemittitur poëma«).

Mailand, Bibl. Ambrosiana, A 57 Inf.; s. XVI.
See also **(*bei* Berthelot Ruelle, p. 56)** above (p. 71).

Zosimus Panopolita: *Excerpta varia.*

Stephanus Alexandrinus: (f. 1) *De sacra divinaque arte auri faciendi.*
Heliodorus:
(f. 37) *Contra Theodosium de philosophorum mystica technica.*
(f. 65v) *Ad Dioscorem.*
Synesius, Cleopatra: (f. 98v) *De mensuris et ponderibus.*
Zosimus Panopolita: (f. 104v) *Liber de virtute et compositione aquarum.*

Mailand, Bibl. Ambrosiana, A 193 Inf.; s. XVI.
See also (***bei*** **Berthelot Ruelle, p. 56)** above (p. 71).

Zosimus Panopolita: *Excerpta varia.*
Stephanus Alexandrinus: (f. 1) *De sacra divinaque arte auri faciendi.*
Heliodorus: (f. 35v) *Contra Theodosium de philosophorum mystica technica.*
Synesius: (f. 64) *Ad Dioscorem.*
Cleopatra: (f. 100v) *De mensuris et ponderibus.*
Zosimus Panopolita: (f. 106v) *Liber de virtute et compositione aquarum.*

Mailand, Bibl. Ambrosiana, C 222 Inf.; s. XIII.

Philo, Herennius: (f. 41v) *De aetatibus hominis.*

Mailand, Bibl. Ambrosiana, D 338 Inf.; s. XV.

Nemesius Emesenus: (f. 1) *De natura hominis.*

Mailand, Bibl. Ambrosiana, D 477 Inf.; s. XVI.

Dioscurides: *Excerpta* (In partem D. notae M. Ant. Maranthae).

Mailand, Bibl. Ambrosiana, E 10 Inf.; s. XI.

Gregorius Nyssenus: (f. 91) *De hominis opificio* (Inc. ⟨γεγονό⟩των διέλαθεν = Migne p. 144 cap. 8).

Mailand, Bibl. Ambrosiana, H 2 Inf.; s. XVI.

Petosiris: (f. 228v) *Epistula ad regem Nechepso* (Inc. Περὶ ἑνὸς ἑκάστου. Expl. ὁ κίνδυνος ἢ οὔ).
Pythagoras: (f. 247) *Prognostica.*
Alexander Rex: (f. 250) *De septem herbarum facultate.*

Mailand, Bibl. Ambrosiana, I 166 Inf.; s. XVII.

Aëtius Amidenus: (f. 62–73) *Excerpta varia.*

Messina, Bibl. S. Salvatoris

Messina, Bibl. S. Salvatoris, 84; s. X–XI.
Now Biblioteca Regioniale Universitaria Giacomo Longo di Messina, S. Salvatore, 84 (*Census*: 137, nr [0681]).
See also **Messina, Universität, 84** below.

Aëtius Amidenus: *Iatricorum libri XVI* (L. I–III p. 63 ed. Ald. *Vgl.* Rühl, Philol. nov. ser. I 581. Olivieri, Studi ital. IX 299–367).

Messina, Universität
Now at the Biblioteca Regionale Universitaria Giacomo Longo di Messina

Messina, Universität, 84; s. –.
Same as **Messina, Bibl. S. Salvatoris, 84** above.
Now Biblioteca Regioniale Universitaria Giacomo Longo di Messina, S. Salvatore, 84.

Oribasius: *Excerpta varia* (Cf. Rühl Philol. N. F. I 577–588).

Mileae

Mileae, Bibl. Mileens., 78; a. 1774.
Now Μηλεαί, Δημόσια Βιβλιοθήκη Μηλεών, 78.

Dioscurides: *De materia medica* (Libri VIII).

Mitylene, Bibl. gymnas.
Now Μυτιλήνη Λέσβου, Βιβλιοθήκη, Πρότυπο Πειραματικό Γενικό Λύκειο Μυτιλήνης του Πανεπιστημίου Αιγαίου

Mitylene, Bibl. Gymnas., 1; a. 1598.

Gregorius Nyssenus: (nr 2) *De hominis opificio*.

Mitylene, Bibl. Gymnas., 33; a. 1774.
= 31 (*Census*: 140, nr [0686]).

Dioscurides: (f. 1–224) *Excerpta*.

Paulus Aegineta: (nr 2. 3. 4) *Excerpta varia* (2: Δίαιτα διὰ τὴν γεροντικὴν ἡλικίαν. 3: ἐπιστολὴ πρὸς Διοκλέα … προφυλακτική. Inc. Ἐπειδή σοι συμβαίνει. 4: περὶ τῶν κενωτικῶν τῆς κεφαλῆς ἀποφλεγματισμῶν τε καὶ ἐρρίνων καὶ διαχιστῶν. μς'. Inc. Τοὺς ἐν τῇ κεφαλῇ χυμούς).

Modena, Bibl. Estense
Now Modena, Biblioteca Estense Universitaria

Modena, Bibl. Estense, 18 (III A 4); s. XV.
Now α.U.9.18 (*Census*: 141, nr [0687]).

Nemesius Emesenus: *De natura hominis*.

Modena, Bibl. Estense, 61 (III B 9); s. XV.
Now α.U.9.4 (*Census*: 141, nr [0689]).

Theophilus: (f. 2) *De urinis*.
Paulus Aegineta: (f. 14) *De succedaneis, ex Galeno*.
Aëtius Amidenus: (f. 29ᵛ) *Excerpta varia* (Frgm. Inc. Ἕπονται δὲ καὶ τοῖς πυρετοῖς ἱδρῶτες. Expl. στοχάσασθαι τοῖς ἀτμοῖς ἐν λουτροῖς).
Theophilus: (f. 31) *Excerpta varia*.

Modena, Bibl. Estense, 109 (II D 10); s. XIV–XV.
Now α.P.5.20 (*Census*: 141, nr [0694]).

Alexander Aphrodisiensis: (f. 3, 24ᵛ) *Problematum physicorum et* medicorum *eclogae. Libri V* (f. 3: L. I et II; Idel. 6, 1–80, 36; f. 24ᵛ: L. III).
Cassius iatrosophistes: (f. 79ᵛ) *Quaestiones medicae et problemata physica* (Ideler I 144, 1–152, 4).

Modena, Bibl. Estense, 115 (II D 16); s. XV.
Now α.P.5.17 (*Census*: 141, nr [0695]).

Theophilus: (f. 9) *De urinis* (Frgm.).
Dioscurides:
(f. 10) *De materia medica*.
(f. 19) *De materia medica*.
(f. 167ᵛ) *De venenis eorumque praecautione et medicatione*.
(f. 175) *De iis, quae virus eiaculantur, animalibus libellus, in quo et de rabioso cane*.
Diocles: (f. 186) *Ad Antigonum regem epistula de tuenda valetitudine*.

Dioscurides: (f. 187) *De mensuris et ponderibus.*

Modena, Bibl. Estense, 135 (II E 2); s. XV.
Now α.T.8.5 (*Census*: 141, nr [0696]).

Alexander Aphrodisiensis: (f. 118) *Problematum physicorum et medicorum eclogae. Libri V* (Inc. Διὰ τί τοὺς ἀνθρώπους. Expl. ὁμοίως δὲ καὶ ἐπὶ νεφελῶν).
Theophylactus Simocatta: (f. 123ᵛ) *Quaestiones naturales.*

Modena, Bibl. Estense, 145 (II E 12); s. XV.
Now α.V.7.17 (*Census*: 141, nr [0697]).

Alexander Aphrodisiensis:
(f. 52) *Problematum physicorum et medicorum eclogae. Libri V* (L. I et II).
(f. 65) *Quarundam difficultatum solutiones* (Περὶ τετραπόδων ἀπορίαι καὶ λύσεις διάφοροι. Τόμος ε', probl. Α'–ΞΓ').
Cassius iatrosophistes: (f. 70) *Quaestiones medicae et problemata physica* (Ideler I 144–151, 37).

Modena, Bibl. Estense, 174 (II F 9); s. XV.
Now α.V.7.6 (*Census*: 142, nr [0699]).

Petosiris:
(f. 262) *Epistula ad regem Nechepso* (Inc. Περὶ τῶν κατακλινομένων ἐν ἀρρωστίαις εὑρήσονται [l. εἰ ῥύσονται]. Expl. ὄργανον ὑπέργειον ἀστρονομικόν. Ed. *im* Catal. cod. astr. IV p. 120 sq.).
(f. 263) *De decubitu infirmorum* (Inc. Ἐὰν ἐν κυριακῇ ἢ τετράδι κατακλιθῇ τις. Expl. ἡ πέμπτη ♃ᵛ. »Post Petosiridis epistulam neque vero sub eius nomine traditur«).
(f. 263) *Organum de vita et morte* (Inc. Μάθε πότε κατεκλίθη ὁ ἄρρωστος. Expl. ζωὴ σκότος ὑπὲρ γῆν. »Post Petosiridis epistulam neque vero sub eius nomine traditur«).

Modena, Bibl. Estense, 210 (III G 6); s. XVI.
Now α.V.6.12 (*Census*: 142, nr [0702]).

Alexander Aphrodisiensis;
(f. 178) *Quarundam difficultatum solutiones* (L. I et II).
(f. 299ᵛ) *Problematum physicorum et medicorum eclogae. Libri V* (*Wie im* Bonon. [2294] [see p. 24]).
Cassius iatrosophistes: (f. 371) *Quaestiones medicae et problemata physica.*

Modena, Bibl. Estense, 240 (III F 17); s. XV–XVI.
Now α.J.6.28 (*Census*: 142, nr [0715]).

Nemesius Emesenus: (f. 111) *De natura hominis* (Expl. καὶ τῆς ἐνεργείας λαμβάνοντες, δέον = Migne 40 p. 601, 5).

Montpellier

Montpellier, Bibliothèque de l'école (*Vgl.* Montfaucon, II p. 1199).
Same as **Berlin, Königl. Bibl., Phillipps. 1536 (ol. Meerm. 231)** above (p. 19) (*Census*: 144, nr [0716]).
= Berlin, Staatsbibliothek zu Berlin – Preussischer Kulturbesitz SBB-PKB, Phill. 1536.

Rufus: *De corporis humani appellationibus*.

Moskau, Synodialbibl.
Now Государственный Исторический Музей (ГИМ), Синодальная Библиотека Московского Патриархата (Gosudarstvennyi Istoricheskii Muzei [GIM], Sinodal'naya Biblioteka Moskovskogo Patriarchata [State Historical Museum [GIM], Synodial Library of Moscow Patriarchate])

Moskau, Synodialbibl. (*Vgl.* Bussemaker *a. a. O.* [= Bussemaker, *Poët. de re phys. et medica rell.*], p. 75).
Now Sinod. 292 (*Census*: 145–146, nr [0721]).
Same as **260** below.

Asclepiades: *Praecepta salubria*.

Moskau, Synodialbibl., 260; a. 1630.
See also **(*Vgl.* Bussemaker *a. a. O.* [= Bussemaker, *Poët. de re phys. et medica rell.*], p. 75)** above.
Now Sinod. 292 (*Census*: 146, nr [0724]).

Oribasius: (f. 254^{v}) *Excerpta varia* (Inc. Εὐεξίας τράπεζαν, εἰ θέλεις, μάθε).

Moskau, Synodialbibl., 436; s. XIII, XIV.
Now Sinod. 298 (*Census*: 147, nr [0728]).

Rufus: (f. 115) *Excerpta varia* (Περὶ τῆς τοῦ πηγάνου χρήσεως. Inc. Πηγάνου οὐδὲν εἰς τὴν ἰατρικὴν χρησιμώτερον).

Moskau, Synodialbibl., 446; s. XV.
= Sinod. 1 (*Census*: 147, nr [0730]).

Alexander Trallianus: (f. 5) *Therapeutica. Libri XII.*

Moskau, Synodialbibl., 464; s. XV.
= Sinod. 51 (*Census*: 147, nr [0731]).

Theophylactus Simocatta: (f. 301) *Versus in Galenum.*

Moskau, Synodialbibl., 466; s. XVI.
= Sinod. 283 (*Census*: 147, nr [0733]).

Herophilus: (f. 20v) *De febricantibus* (Inc. Ὁ δὲ Ἡρ. πυρέσσειν ἀπεφήνατο).

Moskau, Synodialbibl., 468; s. XVI, XVII.
Now Sinod. 508 (*Census*: 147, nr [0735]).

Harpocration: (f. 114) *De facultatibus naturalibus animalium et herbarum et lapidum.*
Aëtius Amidenus: (f. 152) *Excerpta varia* (Π. βοτανῶν κατὰ στοιχεῖον Inc. Ἀργεμὸν βοτάνη ῥίζαν ἔχει).

Moskau, Synodialbibl., 477; a. 1624.
Now Sinod. 506 (*Census*: 147, nr [0736]).

Dioscurides: (f. 8) *Excerpta* (Ἀπὸ τὰ ἰατρικὰ βιβλία τοῦ Δ. μερικὰ εἰς κοινὴν μεταγλωττισθέντα. Inc. Περὶ ἴριδος. Expl. Περὶ σελίνου).

Moskau, Synodialbibl., 498; s. XVI.
Now Sinod. 187 (*Census*: 147, nr [0737]).

Oribasius: (f. 2) *Conspectus ad Eustathium filium. Libri II.*

Moskau, Synodialbibl., 499; s. XVI.
Now Sinod. 188 (*Census*: 148, nr [0738]).

Oribasius: (f. 3) *Ad Eunapium de parabilibus medicamentis. Libri IV.*

München

München, Bibl. August., 542; s. XV.
= Munich, Bayerische Staatsbibliothek, *Monacensis graecus* 542 (*Census*: 151, nr [0739]).

Hermes Trismegistus: (f. 67) *De succis plantarum*.

München, Hof- und Staatsbibliothek
Now München, Bayerische Staatsbibliothek

München, Hof- und Staatsbibliothek (*vgl.* Bussemaker *a. a. O.* [= Bussemaker, Poët. de re phys. et medica rell.]).
= *graecus* 336 (*Census*: 15, nr [0740]).

Asclepiades: *Praecepta salubria*.

[München, Hof- und Staatsbibliothek, Hardt 1 p. 448].
= *graecus* 72 below (p. 86) (*Census*: 151, nr [0742]).

Paulus Nicaeensis: *De cognitione et curatione variorum morborum* (*Wahrscheinlich Irrtum*).

München, Hof- und Staatsbibliothek, graec. 29; s. XVI.

Oribasius: (f. 81) *Medicae collectiones ad Iulianum* (L. VII 2 *und* 13).
Nemesius Emesenus: (f. 108–159. 170^{v}–175^{v}) *De natura hominis* (Expl. ἐπιδέουσιν ἀπαράβατον = 301, 4 Matth.).

München, Hof- und Staatsbibliothek, graec. 39; s. XVI.

Meletius monachus: (f. 1) *De natura hominis* (Inscr. Πόνημα ἐν συνόψει περὶ φύσεως ἀνθρώπου ἐξερανισθὲν καὶ συντεθὲν παρὰ Μελετίου μοναχοῦ ἐκ τῶν τῆς ἐκκλησίας ἐνδόξων καὶ τῶν ἔξω λογάδων καὶ φιλοσόφων. Inc. Τὰ περὶ τῆς τοῦ ἀνθρώπου κατασκευῆς καὶ ἐξ ὅσων ἐστὶ φύσεων. Expl. f. 71 ἐκ τῶν λαμβανομένων τροφῶν. *Darauf folgt, wie zu dem Werke des Meletius gehörig*, περὶ ψυχῆς πρόλογος. Inc. Ὁ περὶ ψυχῆς ὧδε [sic] λόγος οὐ τὸ τί ἐστιν ἡ ψυχή, *vgl.* Med.-Kat. II S. 62. Expl. f. 72^{v} προαίρεσις – ἐπιθυμία, λογικαί – ἄλογοι. *Dahinter wiederum ohne Abtrennung von dem frühern f.* 72^{v}: Περὶ ψυχῆς λόγος δεύτερος. Inc. Ἐπειδὴ δὲ ἐκ ψυχῆς καὶ σώματος συνέστη ὁ ἄνθρωπος. Expl. f. 79^{v} σῶμα δὲ τὴν φράσιν. δόξαν χριστῷ τῷ θεῷ usw. ἀμήν).

München, Hof- und Staatsbibliothek, graec. 69; s. XVI.

Ioannes Zacharias Actuarius:
(f. 1) *De spiritu animali libri II.*
(f. 46) *De methodo medendi Libri VI.*
Paulus Aegineta: (f. 298) *De succedaneis, ex Galeno.*

München, Hof- und Staatsbibliothek, graec. 70; s. XVI.

Diocles: (f. 228) *Ad Antigonum regem epistula de tuenda valetitudine.*
Aretaeus:
(f. 254) *De causis et signis acutorum morborum libri II* (Inc. *wie im* [Berol.] Phillipps. 1531 [see above p. 17]).
(f. 272) *De causis et signis diuturnorum morborum libri II.*
(f. 305) *De curatione acutorum morborum libri II.*

München, Hof- und Staatsbibliothek, graec. 71; a. 1531.

Soranus: (f. 9) *Hippocratis genus et vita secundum Soranum.*
Erotianus: *Vocum Hippocraticarum conlectio*

München, Hof- und Staatsbibliothek, graec. 72; s. XVI.
See also **[Hof- und Staatsbibliothek, Hardt 1 p. 448]** above (p. 85).

Esdras Propheta: *Pro hydropicis et omnibus morbis frigidis.*
Oribasius: (f. 1) *Ad Eunapium de parabilibus medicamentis. Libri IV.*
Aretaeus:
(f. 113) *De causis et signis acutorum morborum libri II* (L. I c. 1–6 desunt).
(f. 129) *De causis et signis diuturnorum morborum libri II.*
(f. 162) *De curatione acutorum morborum libri II.*
(f. 193) *De curatione diuturnorum morborum libri II.*
Lucas: (f. 277) *Compositio salsi intinctus.*

München, Hof- und Staatsbibliothek, graec. 100; s. 1551.

Nemesius Emesenus: (f. 152–170^{v}) *De natura hominis* (*Ergänzung der vorhergehenden Hds.* [Monac. 29] [above p. 85]).

München, Hof- und Staatsbibliothek, graec. 105; s. XVI.

Hermes Trismegistus: (f. 213) *Iatromathematica ad Ammonium Aegyptium.*
Gregorius Theologus: (f. 333 [333^{v}]) *Alatium.*

München, Hof- und Staatsbibliothek, graec. 227; s. XVI.

Damascius: (f. 1) *Expositio in aphorismos Hippocratis. Sectiones VII.*

München, Hof- und Staatsbibliothek, graec. 236; s. XV.

Dioscurides:
(f. 83) *De materia medica* (Sine titulo. Libri VI–IX. *Ist zu streichen*).
(f. 83) *De venenis eorumque praecautione et medicatione* (Πεδακίου Διοσκορίδου Ἀναζαρβέως λόγος ϛ' περὶ δηλητηρίων φαρμάκων καὶ τῆς αὐτῶν προφυλῶν [sic]. Expl. f. 100 τὰς ἀντιδότους ἀναγκαιότατα καὶ γενναιότατα).
(f. 100v–123v) *De iis, quae virus eiaculantur, animalibus libellus, in quo et de rabioso cane* (Inscr. f. 100v praemisso capitum indice: Βιβλίον ζ'ον περὶ ἰοβόλων, ἐν ᾧ καὶ περὶ λυσσῶντος κυνός. Inc. Τὸν μὲν περὶ τῶν ἰοβόλων ζῴων. Expl. f. 112r καὶ τελέως ἀβοήθητα παρασημειούμεθα. Subscr. f. 112v Πεδ. Διοσκ. Ἀναζ. Κιλικίας βιβλίον ἔκδομον [leg. ἔβδομον]: προοίμιον περὶ ἰοβόλων καὶ περὶ σημειώσεως τῶν λυσσοδήκτων. Inscr. f. 112v Πεδ. Διοσκ. Ἀναζ. λόγος ὄγδοος περὶ σημειώσεως τῶν ὑπὸ ἰοβόλων δεδηκμένων [leg. δεδηγμένων]. Inc. Τοῖς δὲ ὑπὸ φαλαγγίων δεδηγμένοις. Expl. f. 118v πρὸς ἕκαστον τῶν ἰοβόλων ἑξῆς ἴδωμεν. Inscr. f. 119 Πεδ. Διοσκ. Ἀναζ. θεραπεῖαι τῶν ὑπὸ ἰοβόλων δεδηγμένων λόγος θ'ος Inc. ⟨Ἐ⟩ν τῇ σημει... περὶ σφικῶν. Expl. f. 123v καὶ οὗτος ὁ θηριακὸς τρόπος. *Die Bücher Z' bis Θ' bilden also zusammen die Schrift* Περὶ ἰοβόλων).

München, Hof- und Staatsbibliothek, graec. 287; s. XIV, XIV ex., XV.

Gregorius Theologus: (f. 1) *Alatium.*
Pythagoras: (f. 135) *Supputationes prognosticae* (Ψῆφος περὶ ζωῆς καὶ θανάτου).

München, Hof- und Staatsbibliothek, graec. 288, s. XIV.

Gregorius Theologus: *Alatium* (Inc. Ὑσσώπου κρητικοῦ).
Ioannes Archiatrus: (f. 7) *Variorum morborum curatio* (Ἑρμηνεία καὶ διδασκαλία καὶ ἐξήγησις τοῦ θαυμασιωτάτου καὶ λογιωτάτου ἀρχιητροῦ τοῦ Γαληνοῦ τοῦ σπεύσαντος εἰς τὸ [sic !] τῶν μορίων πάθη, ἀνίατα καὶ δυσίατα λέγω ἅμα καὶ εὔατα γενέσθαι ὠφέλειαν ἴασιν. Inc. Πρῶτον μὲν καὶ κοινῷ λόγῳ).

München, Hof- und Staatsbibliothek, graec. 308; s. XII.

Splenius philosophus: (f. 223) *De generatione hominis* (Sine auctoris nomine).

München, Hof- und Staatsbibliothek, graec. 362; s. XVI.

Ioannes Zacharias Actuarius: (f. 112) *De urinis libri VII.*

München, Hof- und Staatsbibliothek, graec. 401; s. XVI.

Hermes Trismegistus: (f. 318) *Iatromathematica ad Ammonium Aegyptium* (Inc. mut. κινδυνεῦσας [sic] εἰς χρόνον = Idel. I 431, 36. Expl. mut. κατακλιθῇ τις Κρόνου συνόντος = Id. I 438, 10. »Multis locis discrepat scriptura huius codicis ab editione Ideleri sive Hoeschelii«).

München, Hof- und Staatsbibliothek, graec. 419; s. XIV.

Nemesius Emesenus: (f. 1) *De natura hominis* (Inc. Τὸν ἄνθρωπον ἐκ ψυχῆς νοερᾶς καὶ σώματος ἄριστα κατεσκευάσθαι. Expl. f. 32^{v} τὰ γὰρ φύσει τὰ αὐτὰ παρὰ πᾶσιν = 331, 2 Matth.).

München, Hof- und Staatsbibliothek, graec. 469; s. XIII, XV.
s. XIV (?).
f. 1–50: *nach alter Zählung* φυλλ. ιη'–ϙγ' *am rechten Rande (also vorher die ersten 17 Blätter verloren)*; f. 1–50^{v}: *nach neuerer Zählung am untern Rande, die öfter mehrere Blätter überspringt*; f. 51–55: *nach alter Zählung am rechten Rande* φυλλ. ϙδ'–ϙγ', *nach neuerer am unteren Rande f. 51–55^{v}*; f. 55^{v}: φυλλ. ϙη' *nach alter Zählung am rechten Rande.*

Rufus:

(f. 137–147 [f. 137–147^{v}]) *De medicamentis purgantibus* (*Von derselben Hand vorher* Galenus π. κράσ. κ. δυν. τῶν ἁπλ. φαρμ. *und* Galenus Τίνας δεῖ καθαίρειν καὶ ποίοις καθαρτηρίοις καὶ πότε. *Letzteres Buch hat folg. Subscr.:* ἐνταῦθα τέλος Γαληνοῦ μονοβίβλου, *dann auf derselben Zeile:* ἡ ἀρχὴ Ῥούφου μονοβίβλου. Inc. οὔτε πάντας τοὺς ὁπωσοῦν διακειμένους καθαρτέον. Expl. στήθους καὶ πνεύμονος).

(f. 148–160) *De vesicae renumque affectibus* (*Vielfach zerstört.* Inc. f. 148^{r}. Expl. f. 160^{v} mut. νίτρῳ μετὰ ὄξους ἀνατρίβειν = Dbg. p. 61, 4. *Fortsetzung auf f.* 164^{r}, *bis zum Schlusse des Werkes*).

(f. 161–165) *De satyriasi et gonorrhoea* (»Fragmentum huius opusculi esse censet Daremberg p. XVI sq.«; *Vielfach zerstört.* Inc. f. 164^{v} Τοῦ αὐτοῦ, scil. Ῥούφου, περὶ ... flg. Z. ᾧ τὸ αἰδοῖον *vgl. Anfang des Werkes,* Dbg. p. 64, 1. f. 164^{v} expl. εἰ πρὸς τοῦτο ... = Dbg. p. 67, 1. *Fortsetzung auf f.* 161^{r} ⟨ε⟩ὑρίσκεται · πῶς οὖν = Dbg. p. 67, 2, *und so fort f.* 161. 162 *bis* 163^{v}, *dann f.* 165. Subscr. f. 165^{v} περὶ σατυριασμοῦ ἢ [sic] γονοροί⟨ας⟩).

(f. 161–165) *Excerpta varia* (»Frgm. fortasse ex libello περὶ ἀφροδισίων.« *Vgl.* Daremberg p. XI).

München, Hof- und Staatsbibliothek, graec. 484 (542) (?); s. –.
= (?) *graecus* 489 (*Census*: 155, nr [0764]).

Dioscurides: *Liber agens de experientia medica, de simplicibus et compositis medicamentis, ordine literarum digestus.*

München, Hof- und Staatsbibliothek, graec. 498; s. XIII.

Splenius philosophus: (f. 227) *De generatione hominis* (Sub nomine Ioannis Damasceni).

München, Hof- und Staatsbibliothek, graec. 511; s. XVI.

Muscio: *De morbis mulierum.*

München, Hof- und Staatsbibliothek, graec. 514; s. XIV.
= *graecus* 564 (*Census*: 156, nr [0768]).

Timotheus Gazaeus: (f. 239) *De animalibus quadrupedis physicisque eorum facultatibus* (Frgm.).

München, Hof- und Staatsbibliothek, graec. 521; s. XV.

Diocles: (f. 256v) *Ad Antigonum regem epistula de tuenda valetudine.*

München, Hof- und Staatsbibliothek, graec. 536; s. XV.

Nemesius Emesenus: (f. 1) *De natura hominis* (Inscr. Ἀδαμαντίωνος λόγος κεφαλαιώδης).

München, Hof- und Staatsbibliothek, graec. 551; s. XV.

Lucas: (f. 303) *Compositio salsi intinctus.*

München, Hof- und Staatsbibliothek, graec. 562; s. XVI, XI.

Nemesius Emesenus: (f. 1) *De natura hominis.*

München, Hof- und Staatsbibliothek, graec. 583 (olim Uffenbachianus); a. 1656.
= *graecus* 583 (*Census*: 157, nr [0774]).

Melampus: *De palpitatione divinatio ad regem Ptolemaeum* (Apogr. des Editio Romana).

Neapel, Biblioteca Borbonica
Now Napoli, Biblioteca Nazionale Vittorio Emanuele III

Neapel, Biblioteca Borbonica, I 17; s. XV.
= (?) III D 17 (*Census*: 161, nr [0776]).

Nepualius: (f. 9) *De sympathicis et antipathicis* (Inscr. Τῶν κατὰ ἀντιπάθ. καὶ συμπ.).

Neapel, Biblioteca Borbonica, II C 33; a. 1495.
= II C 32 (*Census*: 162, nr [0777] and 159).
Same as **II C 33 (olim 34)** below. See also **Bibl. di S. Giovanni di Carbonara, 15** below (p. 91).

Splenius philosophus: (f. 7^{v}) *De generatione hominis* (Inscr. Σπλίνου φίλοσ. π. γεν. ἀνθρ. καὶ διαλύσεως).

Neapel, Biblioteca Borbonica, II C 33 (olim 34); a. 1495.
= II C 32 (*Census*: 162, nr [0778]).
Same **as II C 33** above. See also **Bibl. di S. Giovanni di Carbonara, 15** below (p. 91).

Petosiris: (f. 307^{v}) *Epistula ad regem Nechepso* (Inc. Περὶ ἑνὸς ἑκάστου τῶν ὑπ' ἐμοῦ; *vgl. den* Laurent. 86, 14. Expl. ταχέως τελευτήσει).

Neapel, Biblioteca Borbonica, III D 21.
Same as **305 (III D 21)** below.

Aretaeus: *De causis et signis acutorum morborum Libri II.*

Neapel, Biblioteca Borbonica, 304 D III 20; s. XIV.
Now III D 20 (*Census*: 163, nr [0785]).
See also **Bibl. di S. Giovanni di Carbonara, 42** below (p. 92).

Oribasius: *Medicae collectiones ad Iulianum* (L. I–XV).

Neapel, Biblioteca Borbonica, 305 (III D 21); s. XIV.
Same as **III D 21** above (*Census*: 163, nr [0786]).
Now III D 21.

Aretaeus:
De causis et signis acutorum morborum libri II.
De curatione acutorum morborum libri II.
De causis et signis diuturnorum morborum libri II.

De curatione diuturnorum morborum libri II.

Neapel, Biblioteca Borbonica, 306 (III D 22); s. XIII.
Now III D 22 (*Census*: 163, nr [0787]).

Paulus Aegineta: *Epitomae medicae libri septem* (L. I–III lacunos.).

Neapel, Biblioteca Borbonica, 307 (III D 23); s. XV.
Now III D 23 (*Census*: 163, nr [0788]).

Dioscurides: (f. 1) *De facile parabilibus tam simplicibus quam compositis medicamentis libri II.*
Mercurius monachus: (f. 137) *De pulsibus.*
Ioannes Zacharias Actuarius: (f. 139) *Tractatus de urinis, qui ex Avicenna translatus dicitur in graecam linguam a Christodulo, in ordinem redactus ab Actuario Zacharia.*

Neapel, Biblioteca dei Gerolamini Now Napoli, Biblioteca statale oratoriana del Monumento nazionale dei Girolamini

Neapel, Bibl. dei Gerolamini, XXII.1; s. XIV, XV.
Now Biblioteca statale oratioriana del Monumento nazionale dei Girolamini, Pil. XXII. nr I (*Census*: 163, nr [0789]).
See also **Bibl. Oratoriana, 152 (Pil. XXII nr 1)** below (p. 92).

Meletius monachus: (f. 157^{v}–160^{v}) *De natura hominis* (Frgm. Μερικαί τινες παρεκβολαὶ ἐκ τοῦ περὶ φύσεως ἀνθρώπου πονήματος τοῦ ... Μελετίου. Inc. Οὗτός φησὶν ἄνθρωπός ἐστι ζῷον λογικόν. Expl. μετὰ τὴν γαστέρα κεῖται).
Diocles: (f. 174) *Ad Antigonum regem epistula de tuenda valetitudine.*
Aëtius Amidenus: (f. 176) *Excerpta varia* (Ποδαγρικαὶ θεραπεῖαι πρόχειροι. Inc. Κένωσις διὰ φλεβοτομίας. Expl. ἐπίθες).

Neapel, Bibliotheca di S. Giovanni di Carbonara

Neapel, Bibl. di S. Giovanni di Carbonara, 15; s. XIV.
Same as **II C 33, II C 33 (olim 34)** (p. 90) (*Census*: 163, nr [0790]).
Now Biblioteca Nazionale Vittorio Emanuele III, II C 32.

Hermes Trismegistus: *Excerpta varia.*

Neapel, Bibl. di S. Giovanni di Carbonara, 42; s. XV.
Same as **304 D III 20** above (p. 90) (*Census*: 164, nr [0792]).
Now Biblioteca Nazionale Vittorio Emanuele III, III D 20.

Oribasius: *Medicae collectiones ad Iulianum* (L. I–XV).

Neapel, Bibliotheca Oratoriana

Neapel, Bibl. Oratoriana, 152 (Pil. XXII nr 1); s. XIV–XV.
Same as **Bibl. dei Gerolamini, XXII.1** above (p. 91) *Census*: 164, nr [0794]).
Now Biblioteca statale oratoriana del Monumento nazionale dei Girolamini, Pil. XXII. nr I.

Diocles: *Ad Antigonum regem epistula de tuenda valetitudine.*
Meletius monachus: *De natura hominis* (Frgm. Moschopuli Excerpta).

Orléans

Orléans, Bibl. communale, 1032; s. XVII.
Now Médiathèque.

Hermes Trismegistus: (p. 121) *Excerpta varia* (Tabula smaragdina περὶ χημείας).

Oxford, Bibl. Aedis Christi
Now Oxford, Christ Church Library

Oxford, Bibl. Aedis Christi, 81; s. XVII.

Aretaeus:
De causis et signis acutorum morborum libri II.
De causis et signis diuturnorum morborum libri II.
De curatione acutorum morborum libri II.
De curatione diuturnorum morborum libri II (fine mut.).

Oxford, Bibl. Bodleiana

Oxford, Bibl. Bodleiana, – (Puschm. I p. 90).
= Bodleian Library, Ms. D'Orville 34 (*Census*: 168–169, nr [0802]).

Alexander Trallianus: *Epistula de lumbricis.*

Oxford, Bibl. Bodleiana, *e 19 [31.528]*.
= MS. Gr. class. e. 19. (*Census*: 169, nr [0803]).

H. C. Conybeares Kopie und Photographien (of manuscript Edschmiadzin nr. ? above [p. 32]).

Oxford, Bibl. Bodleiana, Baroccian. 50; s. XI.

Timotheus Gazaeus: (f. 46) *De animalibus quadrupedis physicisque eorum facultatibus.*
Aelianus: (f. 386 b) *Epistula* (»An Aeliani?« Coxe).

Oxford, Bibl. Bodleiana, Baroccian. 82; s. XV.

Nemesius Emesenus: (f. 156) *De natura hominis* (Expl. mutil. καὶ μηδένα edit. Oxon. 1671 p. 305, 13).

Oxford, Bibl. Bodleiana, Baroccian. 88; s. XV–XVI, XV (XVI), XVI.

Athenaeus: *Synopsis de urinis.*
Hermes Trismegistus: *Excerpta varia* (Inc. Πηγάνου φύλλων ξηρῶν, παιωνίας, ὀριγάνου, ὀποπάνακος, καρποβαλσάμου).
Paulus Aegineta: *Epitomae medicae libri septem* (L. II 1–5).
Aëtius Amidenus: *Iatricorum libri XVI* (L. I. II 12. 82. 84 ss. 193 alia).
Leo: (f. 18) *Excerpta* (Περὶ μελαγχολίας et alia capita de Leone desumpta. *Vgl.* Ermerins, Anecd. med. gr. *a. a. O.*).
Paulus Italus, Athenaeus, Ioannes Tzetzes: (f. 47) *Prognostica/Excerpta* (Ἱπποκρ. διδασκάλου καὶ Γαλ. σοφοῦ καὶ Παύλου Ἰτάλου καὶ Ἀθηναίου ῥήτορος καὶ Ἰωάννου Τζέτζου διάγνωσις περὶ ἰαλίων [l. ὑαλίων] ἀρρώστων καὶ τελευτῆς ἀνθρώπων. Inc. Τὸ α'. ἄσπρον. Expl. σημαίνει καὶ θάνατον).
Palladius: (f. 51v–54v) *Stephani philosophi vel Palladii synopsis de febribus* (Expl. διαφοραὶ τῶν πυρετῶν. ἁλμυρώδεας δὲ λέγει τοὺς συμβαίνοντας τοῖς ὑπερκοπωθεῖσιν, ὡς γινομένου ξηροτέρου τοῦ δέρματος οἷον ἐπὶ τῶν ταριχευομένων σωμάτων. Verba ἁλμυρώδεας κτλ. apud Idelerum desunt).

Aëtius Amidenus: (f. 109^{v}) *Iatricorum libri XVI* (L. V praeter capp. 121–131. L. VI praeter capp. 1–3 partim, quorum loco capp. l. III praeter 1–9. 162–170. 174. 175. 179–185).
Asclepiades, Dioscurides: (f. 164 b) *Excerpta varia* (Ἐκ τῶν Ἀσκληπιάδου καὶ Διοσκορίδου περὶ ἀναπνοῆς / δυ⟨σπνοίας⟩).

Oxford, Bibl. Bodleiana, Baroccian. 94; s. XV.

Nemesius Emesenus: (f. 43) *De natura hominis* (Frgm. Liber Nemesii ..., in epitomam redactus, forsan ab Andrea Dono).

Oxford, Bibl. Bodleiana, Baroccian. 111; s. XV.

Stephanus Atheniensis: (f. 122) *Excerpta varia* (Γυναῖκα ὁμολογῆσαι, ὑπὸ πόσων ἀνδρῶν ἐμιδύθη κτλ.).

Oxford, Bibl. Bodleiana, Baroccian. 131; s. XIV, XIV in.

Meletius monachus: (f. 1) *De natura hominis* (Περὶ τῆς τοῦ ἀνθρώπου κατασκευῆς).
Alexander Aphrodisiensis: (f. 62 b) *Quarundam difficultatum solutiones.*
Orpheus: (f. 175^{v}) *De lapidibus.*
Alexander Aphrodisiensis: (f. 404 b–405) *Problematum physicorum et medicorum eclogae. Libri V* (Frgm.).

Oxford, Bibl. Bodleiana, Baroccian. 150; s. XV, XV in.

Iustus: *Excerpta* (Ἀντίδοτος ἡ ἱερὰ Ἰούστου πρὸς κεφαλαγίαν).
Nicolaus Myrepsus: *Excerpta* (Inc. Ἀντίδοτος Ἀλεξανδρεία).
Philo: *Excerpta varia* (Ἀντίδοτος ἡ Φίλωνος, ληφθεῖσα περὶ [l. παρὰ ?] τοῦ φιλοσόφου).
Theodoretus: *Antidota.*
Lucas: (f. 1) *Compositio salsi intinctus.*
Logadius: (f. 3 b) *Excerpta* (*Wie im* Athous [Βιβλ. Μον. Ἰβήρων 4271.151]) (see p. 8).
Archigenes: (f. 3 b) *Excerpta varia* (Ἀντίδοτος ἱερά).
Esdras Propheta: (f. 5 b) *Antidotus Esdrae.*
Syncellus: (f. 5 b) *Excerpta* (Ἀντίδοτος ἡ βασιλική).
Herophilus Sophista: (f. 14^{v}) *De alimentis, quae singulis mensibus sumenda aut vitanda sunt* (»Valde differt ab Ideleri editione«).
Lucas: (f. 18) *Compositio salsi intinctus.*
Herophilus Sophista: (f. 18^{v}) *De alimentorum facultatibus* (Expl. τὰ κητώδη πλὴν τῆς ὕσκας ... καὶ περιττωματικά.» Fragmentum, ed. ab Ideler p. 257–281

sub titulo Ἀνωνύμου περὶ χυμῶν, βρωμάτων καὶ πομάτων § 46 sqq., des. p. 281 in cap. Περὶ τῶν ἐκ τῶν ζῴων τροφῆς δυνάμεων. V. huius cod. § 12 et cod. Vindob. nr 28 [below p. 182]«. Vgl. Daremberg, Not. et Extr. I p. 21 sq.).

Oribasius: (f. 20v) *Excerpta varia* (Περὶ ἁπλῶν φαρμάκων κράσεων καὶ μίξεων ὑγιεινῶν κτηνῶν ὁμοῦ καὶ πτηνῶν τῆς ἄγρας κτέ. Inc. Ἐν ἀγρῷ εἰς ἕνα τόπον. Expl. χυλὸς σὺν οἴνῳ ἐγχυματιζόμενος).

Esdras Propheta: (f. 32v) *Antidotus Esdrae.*

Gregorius Theologus: (f. 32v) *Alatium.*

Syncellus: (f. 32 b) *Excerpta* (Ἀντίδοτος).

Dioscurides: (f. 41v) *Liber agens de experientia medica, de simplicibus et compositis medicamentis, ordine literarum digestus.*

Athenaeus: (f. 48v) *De remediis ordine alphabetico* (»Non pauca congruunt cum remediorum collectione sub Dioscoridis et Stephani nomine tradita«. Daremberg, Not. et Extr. I 37).

Alexander Sophista: (f. 67v) *De sacrarum herbarum temperamentis.*

Dioscurides, **Oribasius**, **Porphyrius**, **Paulus Aegineta, Magnus Emesenus**, **Archigenes**: (f. 77) *Excerpta varia* (Pauca quaedam de simplicibus ex Dioscoride, Oribasio, Porphyrio, Paulo, Magno et Archigene).

Oxford, Bibl. Bodleiana, Baroccian. 171; s. XV in.

Nicolaus Myrepsus: (f. 8) *De compositione medicamentorum, alphabetice* (Medicamentum. *Vgl.* Medicae artis principes ed. Stephanus, col. 408).

Oxford, Bibl. Bodleiana, Baroccian. 173; s. XII, XIII.

Moschion: (f. 349) *Praecepta vitae.*

Oxford, Bibl. Bodleiana, Baroccian. 204; s. XV in., XV.

Erotianus: *Vocum Hippocraticarum conlectio.*

Theophilus: (f. 1) *Commentarius in Hippocratis aphorismos* (Initium solum).

Soranus: (f. 8) *Hippocratis genus et vita secundum Soranum.*

Oxford, Bibl. Bodleiana, Baroccian. 216; s. –.

Dioscurides: (f. 108 b) *De mensuris et ponderibus.*

Oxford, Bibl. Bodleiana, Baroccian. 220; s. XIII.

Heraclius: (f. 47v) *Versus politici.*

Oxford, Bibl. Bodleiana, Baroccian. 224; s. XV in., XV.

Oribasius: (f. 1) *Medicae collectiones ad Iulianum* (Frgm. *Wie im* Monac. 29 [above p. 85]).
Paulus Aegineta: (f. 2ᵛ) *Excerpta varia* (*Wie im* Bonon. 3636. f. 61ᵛ [above p. 26]).
Lucas: (f. 21 b) *Compositio salsi intinctus.*
Paulus Aegineta:
(f. 21ᵛ) *Excerpta varia* (Ἄλειμμα πρὸς ῥαγάδας χειρῶν καὶ ποδῶν, πρὸς δὲ τὰς γινομένας ἐν αὐτοῖς ἐγκαύσεις ἀπὸ δὲ τοῦ προσομιλῆσαι χιόνι ἢ ἀνέμῳ χειμερίῳ. Expl. τὸ ζάμβακα καὶ τὸ νάρδον).
(f. 21ᵛ) *Epitomae medicae libri septem* (L. V 1–47).
Africanus: (f. 50ᵛ) *Ex Africani Cestis cestum XIII cap. 22: De purgantibus simplicibus* (Inc. Κυκλαμίνου χυλός. Expl. μυχθεὶς καὶ ποθείς).
Diocles: (f. 50ᵛ) *Ad Antigonum regem epistula de tuenda valetitudine.*

Oxford, Bibl. Bodleiana, Baroccian. 2304; s. –.
= ? Oxford, Bodleian Library, MS. Roe 15 below (p. 100), or Paris, Bibliothèque nationale de France, *graecus* 2304 below (p. 130) (*Census*: 174, nr [0830]).

Ioannes Zacharias Actuarius: *De spiritu animali libri II.*

Oxford, Bibl. Bodleiana, Canonician. 1; s. XVI.

Aëtius Amidenus: (f. 70) *Excerpta varia* (Π. τροφῶν δυνάμεων. Inc. Χρὴ δὲ ὥσπερ τι καὶ ἄλλον. Expl. πρὸς εἴκοντας εὔχυμον γενά [?]).

Oxford, Bibl. Bodleiana, Canonician. 56; s. XVI.

Nemesius Emesenus: (f. 55) *De natura hominis.*

Oxford, Bibl. Bodleiana, Canonician. 109; s. XV ex.

Aëtius Amidenus: *Iatricorum libri XVI* (L. IX–XVI 17. *Nach Zervos Apogr. des Parisin. 2191* [below p. 118]).

Oxford, Bibl. Bodleiana, Is. Casauboni Advers. 27.
Now MS. Casaubon 27 (*Census*: 175, nr [0838]).

Dioscurides: (f. 145. 146) *Excerpta* (Nonnulla ex D. Inc. Ἡ βίβλος περιέχει).

Oxford, Bibl. Bodleiana, Laud. 58 (nunc 59; Bodl. 708); s. XV.
= MS. Laud Gr. 59 (*Census*: 176, nr [0840]).

Athenaeus: *Synopsis de urinis* (»Σημειώσεις οὔρων. Inc. iisdem fere verbis atque opus [Oxon.] Barocc. 88 [above p. 93] traditum. Des. πλευρῖτιν σημαίνει. Est pars operis sub Athenaei nomine traditi [v. Barocc. 88 § 4]; exstat etiam Paris. gr. 2239. f. 160«. *Vgl.* Daremberg Not. et Extr. I 62).
Rufus: (f. 375) *De vesicae renumque affectibus*.

Oxford, Bibl. Bodleiana, Laudian. 62 (Bodl. 747); s. XVI.
Now MS. Laud Gr. 62 (*Census*: 176, nr [0841]).

Ioannes Zacharias Actuarius: *De methodo medendi libri VI*:
(f. 1) L. IV. V.
(f. 95) L. VI c. 8 ss. Inscr. Γαλ. Π. ἐμπλάστρων.

Oxford, Bibl. Bodleiana, Laudian. C 60 (Bodl. 749); s. XVI.
Now MS. Laud Gr. 60 (*Census*: 177, nr [0849]).

Aëtius Amidenus: (f. 1) *Iatricorum libri XVI* (L. IX–XII 49 τικτῶν).

Oxford, Bibl. Bodleiana, Miscell. –; s. XV.
Now MS. Rawl. G. 94 (*Census*: 178, nr [0850]).

Diocles: *Ad Antigonum regem epistula de tuenda valetitudine.*

Oxford, Bibl. Bodleiana, Miscell. 20; s. XIV.
Now MS. Auct. E. 1. 6 (*Census*: 178, nr [0851]).

S. Basilius: (f. 302) *De hominis generatione. Libri III.*
Gregorius Nyssenus: (f. 321v) *De hominis opificio.*

Oxford, Bibl. Bodleiana, Miscell. 69; s. XI (?).
Now MS. Auct. E. 5. 4 (*Census*: 178, nr [0852]).

Nemesius Emesenus: (f. 23 b) *De natura hominis* (In capita 58 distributus. De hominis opificio).

Oxford, Bibl. Bodleiana, Miscell. 130; s. XVII.
Now MS. Auct. F. inf. 2. 1 (*Census*: 178, nr [0853]).

Synesius: (p. 330) *De insomniis.*

Oxford, Bibl. Bodleiana, Miscell. 162; s. XV.
Now MS. Rawl. G. 122 (*Census*: 178, nr [0855]).

Nemesius Emesenus: *De natura hominis*.

Oxford, Bibl. Bodleiana, Miscell. 189; s. XV.
Now MS. Auct. T. 1. 11 (*Census*: 178, nr [0856]).

Aëtius Amidenus: (f. 1) *Iatricorum libri XVI* (Frgm. Tabula cap. L. IX cum prioribus versib. capitis I).

Oxford, Bibl. Bodleiana, Miscell. 211; s. XV.
Now MS. Auct. T. 2. 11 (*Census*: 178, nr [0858]).
See also **Miscell. 211 (Auct. T II 11)** below.

Epiphanius: (f. 73) *De mensuris et ponderibus* (Inc. Κόρος σίτου μόδια λ').

Oxford, Bibl. Bodleiana, Miscell. 211 (Auct. T II 11); s. XV.
Same as **Miscell. 211** above.
= MS. Auct. T. 2. 11 (*Census*: 178, nr [0859]).

Epiphanius: (f. 73–78^{v}) *De mensuris et ponderibus I*.

Oxford, Bibl. Bodleiana, Miscell. 212; s. XVI.
= MS. Auct. T. 2. 12 (*Census*: 178–179, nr [0860]).
See also **Miscell. 212 (Auct. T II 12)** below.

Epiphanius: (f. 87) *De mensuris et ponderibus* (Frgm.).

Oxford, Bibl. Bodleiana, Miscell. 212 (Auct. T II 12); s. XVI.
Same as **Miscell. 212** above.
= MS. Auct. T. 2. 12 (*Census*: 179, nr [0861]).

Epiphanius: (f. 87–97^{v}) *De mensuris et ponderibus I*.

Oxford, Bibl. Bodleiana, Miscell. 241; s. XV.
Now MS. Auct. T. 4. 3 (*Census*: 179, nr [0862]).
See also **Miscell. 241. Auct. T IV 3** below, and **Verona, Bibl. Capitolare, 57 *bei* Montfaucon** (p. 176).

Paulus Aegineta: (f. 182) *De succedaneis, ex Galeno*.

Oxford, Bibl. Bodleiana, Miscell. 241. Auct. T IV 3; s. XV.
Same as **Miscell. 241** above.
= MS. Auct. T. 4. 3 (*Census*: 179, nr [0863]).

Ioannes Zacharias Actuarius: (f. 8) *De urinis libri VII.*

Oxford, Bibl. Bodleiana, Miscell. 278; a. 1780.
Now MS. Auct. T. 5. 16 (*Census*: 179, nr [0864]).

Herophilus Sophista: (p. 8. 22. 25–30. 39–54) *De alimentis, quae singulis mensibus sumenda aut vitanda sunt* (»The fragment on p. 8 is taken from codd. 396 and 985 [pp. 107, 108 below], the rest of the treatise from cod. 396 of the Paris library«).
Neophytus Prodromenus: (p. 135) *Remediorum collectio alphabetica.*

Oxford, Bibl. Bodleiana, d'Orvillian. X 1. 1. 3; s. XV ex.
Now MS. D'Orville 3 (*Census*: 179, nr [0865]).

Oribasius: (f. 1) *Conspectus ad Eustathium filium. Libri II.*
Erotianus: (f. 166) *Vocum Hippocraticarum conlectio.*

Oxford, Bibl. Bodleiana, d'Orvillian. X 1. 4. 3; *nach* 1500.
Now MS. D'Orville 105 (*Census*: 179, nr [0866]).

Nemesius Emesenus: *De natura hominis* (Expl. τὸ δὲ ἀντικείμενον ἀδύνατον).

Oxford, Bibl. Bodleiana, d'Orvillian. X 2. 6. 2 (= 432); s. –.
Now MS. D'Orville 432 (*Census*: 179, nr [0868]).

Nemesius Emesenus: *De natura hominis* (»*A copy of the 1671 Oxford edition, with a collation of a ms. by J. P. d'Orville*«).

Oxford, Bibl. Bodleiana, Roe 14; s. XV.
See also **Roe 14 (Bodl. 260)** below.

Aëtius Amidenus: (f. 86) *Iatricorum libri XVI* (L. V 140 inc. Ὀξύμελι. expl. κεκτημένων).
Esdras Propheta: (f. 280) *Antidotus Esdrae.*
Aëtius Amidenus: (f. 282) *Iatricorum libri XVI* (L. XII).

Oxford, Bibl. Bodleiana, Roe 14 (Bodl. 260); s. XV.
Same as **Roe 14** above.
= MS. Roe 14 (*Census*: 180, nr [0871]).

Theophilus: (f. 87ᵛ) *Commentarius in Hippocratis aphorismos* (= Dtz. II 245–543 ἴαμα).
Meletius monachus: (f. 210) *De natura hominis.*

Oxford, Bibl. Bodleiana, Roe 15 (Bodl. 261); s. XV, XV ex.
= MS. Roe 15 (*Census*: 180, nr [0872]).
See also **Baroccian. 2304** (possibly) above (p. 96).

Meletius monachus: (f. 1) *De natura hominis.*
Theophilus:
(f. 90ᵛ) *De urinis.*
(f. 97ᵛ) *De alvi excrementis.*
Alexander Rex: (f. 103) *De septem herbarum facultate.*
Ioannes Zacharias Actuarius:
(f. 105) *De urinis libri VII.*
(f. 184) *De spiritu animali libri II.*
(f. 218) *De methodo medendi libri VI.*

Padua, Bibl. Joann. Rhodii

Padua, Bibl. Joann. Rhodii.
Verbleib unbekannt.
Now Padova, Biblioteca del Seminario, 194 (*Census*: 190, nr [0889]).

Dioscurides:
Opera varia (D. graece).
Liber agens de experientia medica, de simplicibus et compositis medicamentis, ordine literarum digestus (D. et Stephani Ath. De pharmacis ordine literarum).

Padua, Bibl. Joann. Rhodii.
Verbleib unbekannt.
Now Padova, Biblioteca del Seminario, 194 (*Census*: 192, nr [0898]).

Stephanus Atheniensis: *Dioscoridis et Stephani Atheniensis de pharmacis ordine literarum.*

Padua, Bibl. Joann. Rhodii.
Verbleib unbekannt.
Same as **Kopenhagen, Bibl. Univ., e donatione variorum fol. 29** above (p. 57).
= København, Det Kongelige Bibliotek, e don. var., 29, 2° (*Census*: 192, nr [0899]).

Stephanus Atheniensis: *Enarratio Galeni de methodo medendi ad Glauconem librorum.*

Padua, Bibl. S. Joannis in Viridario

Padua, Bibl. S. Joannis in Viridario, ad dextr. plut. 16.
Verbleib unbekannt.
It was Holkham nr. 283 above (p. 54) and it is now Oxford, Bodleian Library, Holkham Gr. 108 (*Census*: 192, nr [0901]).

Aëtius Amidenus: *Iatricorum libri XVI.*

Padua, Bibl. S. Joannis in Viridario, ad dextr. plut. XVI.
Verbleib unbekannt.
Now Venezia, Biblioteca Nazionale San Marco, *App. gr.* V.1 (coll. 834) below (p. 174) (*Census*: 193, nr [0902]).

Oribasius: *Opera.*

Palermo, Biblioteca nazionale
Now Palermo, Biblioteca centrale della Regione siciliana «Alberto Bombace»

Palermo, Biblioteca nazionale, IV H 8; s. XV.

Alexander Aphrodisiensis: (f. 85v–125) *Problematum physicorum et medicorum eclogae. Libr IV*).

Palermo, Biblioteca nazionale, XIII C 3; s. –, XVI.

Ioannes Zacharias Actuarius: *Tractatus de urinis, qui ex Avicenna translatus dicitur in graecam linguam a Christodulo, in ordinem redactus ab Actuario Zacharia.*
Ioannes Episcopus Prisdianensis: (f. 85–94v) *Collectanea de urinis* (Expl. ἀπαρτίζομεν τὴν διδασκαλίαν).
Theophilus: (f. 96–119v) *De urinis* (Inscr. Σχόλια εἰς τὰ π. οὔρων).

Stephanus Ἀρχιατρὸς τῶν Μαγγάνων: (f. 914^{v}–915^{v}) *Excerpta varia* (Ἀποφλεγματισμὸς ἐαρινὸς κατασπῶν τὰ ἐν τῷ κρανίῳ φλέγματα καὶ χυμούς. Inc. Ὑσσώπου ὄγγ. δ'. Expl. καὶ ὅταν γένηται χλιαρὸν χρῶ. *Vgl.* Daremberg, Not. et Extr. I 33).
Aëtius Amidenus: *Iatricorum libri XVI*:
(f. 940–951^{v}) Frgm. Inscr. Ἐκ τῶν Γαλ. προοίμιον περὶ τῶν δ' τάξεων ἑκάστου γένους τῶν ἁπλῶν φαρμάκων.
(f. 956–1047) Frgm. De plantis ord. alph. Inc. Ἀκαλήφη. Expl. ἀδίκτος ἐστίν.

Paris, Bibl. regia

Paris, 2 Parisini regii *bei Migne* (= Migne, Patrol. gr. 32 p. 684 ff. Ep. 189).
= Paris, Bibliothèque nationale de France, *graecus* 506 and *graecus* 971 (*Census*: 194–195, nrs [0907] and [0908], respectively).

S. Basilius: *Ad Eusthatum medicum de obiectionum haereticorum solutione.*

[Paris, B. R. 349; s. –].
= ? Paris, Bibliothèque nationale de France, *graecus* 2510 below (p. 135) (*Census*: 195–196, nr [0910]).

Lucas: (f. 156) *Compositio salsi intinctus.*

Paris, Bibl. de la ville de Paris/Bibl. de Paris

Paris, Bibl. de la ville de Paris, 12; s. XV.
= Paris, Bibliothèque Mazarine, 4461 below (p. 104) (*Census*: 196–197, nr [0911]).

Dioscurides: (f. 104) *Metaphrasis in Nicandri Theriaca et Alexipharmaca.*

Paris, Bibl. de la ville de Paris, 58; s. XVI–XVII.
= Paris, Bibliothèque Interuniversitaire de Santé – BIU Santé, MS 2105 (*Census*: 197, nr [0912]).

Aëtius Amidenus: *Iatricorum libri XVI* (L. IX–XVI).
Africanus: (f. 609) *De ponderibus et mensuris.*

Paris, Bibl. de Paris, 42; s. XVI.
= Paris, Bibliothèque Sainte-Geneviève, 3394: (*Census*: 198, nr [0914]).

Nemesius Emesenus: (f. 131^{v}) *De natura hominis* (Excerpta varia, ed. Oxon. 1671 capp. 39–41. 29–34. 42. 44. 35. 38).

Paris, Bibl. de Paris, 57; s. XVII.
= Paris, Bibliothèque Interuniversitaire de Santé – BIU Santé, MS 44 (*Census*: 198, nr [0915]).
Same as the following four items below: **Bibl. Facult. Méd., nr.** ?; **Bibl. Facult. Med., 14**; **Bibl. Facult. Medic. 14**; **Facult. Med., 14 (ol. Bibl. de Paris 57)**; and possibly also **Facult. Med., Facult. Med., –**; and **Faculté de Méd.**

Oribasius: (f. 18) *Medicae collectiones ad Iulianum* (L. XLVIII).

Paris, Bibl. Facult. Méd. (Med.) / Faculté de Méd. / Faculté de Médecine. Now Paris, Bibliothèque Interuniversitaire de Santé – BIU Santé

Paris, Facult. Med.
Possibly same as **Bibl. Facult Med. 14 (ol. Bibl. de Paris 57)** and **Paris Faculté de Méd.** below, and also below.
= ? 44 (*Census*: 199, nr [0918]).

Anon. (fort. Actuar.): *De urinis libri VII.*

Paris, Facult. Med., –; s. –.
Possibly same as **Bibl. Facult Med. 14 (ol. Bibl. de Paris 57)** and **Paris Faculté de Méd.** below, and also above.
= ? MS 44 (*Census*: 198, nr [0917]).

Oribasius: *Excerpta varia* (De fracturis fragmenta).

Paris, Facult. Med., 14 (ol. Bibl. de Paris 57); s. XVII.
Same as **Bibl. Facult Med.** above.
= MS 44 (*Census*: 199, nr [0921]).

Oribasius: (f. 18) *Excerpta varia* (De ligamentis et machinamentis chirurgicis, ex Heraclide Ephesio [lib. 48]).
Rufus: (f. 58) *De corporis humani appellationibus*.

Paris, Facult. Méd., 145 (ol. Bibl. de Paris 59); a. 1841–43.
= MS 5112 (*Census*: 199–200, nr [0923]).

Oribasius: *Conspectus ad Eustathium filium. Libri II* (*Apographon des* Parisin. 2188 [below p. 118]).

Paris, Faculté de Méd.
Possibly same as **Bibl. Facult Medic. 14** above.
= ? MS 44 (*Census*: 198, nr [0916]).

Apollonius Citiensis: *Commentarius in Hippocratis de articulis, libri III* (*vgl.* Dietz, Schol. in Hipp. et Gal. I prf. p. XI): II.15.

Paris, Faculté de Médecine, 76; s. XVI–XVII.
= MS 2105 (*Census*: 199, nr [0922]).

Aëtius Amidenus: (f. 1) *Iatricorum libri XVI* (L. IX–XVI).

Paris, Bibl. Mazarine

Paris, Bibl. Mazarine, 4461; s. XV.
See also **Bibl. de la ville de Paris, 12** above (p. 102).

Dioscurides: (f. 104) *Metaphrasis in Nicandri Theriaca et Alexipharmaca*.

Paris, Bibl. Nationale, Coislin. Now Paris, Bibliothèque nationale de France, Coisliniani

Paris, Bibl. Nationale, Coislin. *bei Migne* [= Migne, Patrol. gr. 32 p. 684 ff. Ep. 189].
= 237 (*Census*: 200, nr [0925]).

S. Basilius: *Ad Eusthatum medicum de obiectionum haereticorum solutione*.

Paris, Bibl. Nationale, Coislin., 8; s. X.

Paulus Aegineta: *Epitomae medicae libri septem*:
(f. 1–283)»Frgmta. l. III, sine auctor. nom. trad.«.
(f. 1) = ed. Aldina venetiis 1528, fol. 26^{v}, lin. 4 – fol. 27^{r} l. 12.
(f. 283) = ed. Ald. fol. 29^{r}, l. 10 – fol. 29^{v}, l. 36.

Paris, Bibl. Nationale, Coislin., 78; s. XI.

Ioannes Chrysostomus: (f. 199) *De adversa valetudine et medicis.*

Paris, Bibl. Nationale, Coislin., 79; s. XI–XII.

Ioannes Chrysostomus: (f. 79) *De adversa valetudine et medicis.*

Paris, Bibl. Nationale, Coislin., 115; s. XII.

Nemesius Emesenus: (f. 131^{v}. 170^{v}) *De natura hominis* (Frgm.).

Paris, Bibl. Nationale, Coislin., 120; s. X.

Nemesius Emesenus: (f. 99. 116^{v}) *De natura hominis* (Frgm.).

Paris, Bibl. Nationale, Coislin., 123, f. A; s. X.

Paulus Aegineta: (f. A [*vor* f. 1]) *Epitomae medicae libri septem* (= ed. Ald. fol. 79^{r}, l. 38 – fol. 80^{r}, l. 18).

Paris, Bibl. Nationale, Coislin., 158; s. XVI.

Hermes Trismegistus: *Kyranides* (L. I, A-Y).
Harpocration: (f. 80) *De facultatibus naturalibus animalium et herbarum et lapidum* (Frgm. De lapidibus, plantis A-Y).
Kyranus: (f. 80) *Lexicon de lapidibus, plantis etc.* (A-Y).

Paris, Bibl. Nationale, Coislin., 168; a. 1355.

Paulus Aegineta: (f. 1) *Epitomae medicae libri septem.*

Paris, Bibl. Nationale, Coislin., 228; s. XI–XIV.

Gregorius Nyssenus: (f. 62) *De hominis opificio.*

Paris, Bibl. Nationale, Coislin., 229; s. X–XII.
Now Москва, Научная Библиотека Московского Государственного Университета Имени М. В. Ломоносова (МГУ), гр., 1 (Moskva, Nauchnaia Biblioteka Moskovskogo Gosudarstvennogo Universiteta Imeni M. V. Lomonosova [MGU] – Research Library, Lomonosov Moscow State University [MSU]) (*Census*: 204, nr [0940]).

Gregorius Nyssenus: (f. 83^{v}) *De hominis opificio.*

Paris, Bibl. Nationale, Coislin., 235; s. X–XI.

Gregorius Nyssenus: (f. 121) *De hominis opificio* (fine mutil.).

Paris, Bibl. Nationale, Coislin., 259; a. 1056.

Nemesius Emesenus: (f. 128) *De natura hominis* (Frgm.).

Paris, Bibl. Nationale, Coislin., 294; s. XII.

Nemesius Emesenus: (f. 18) *De natura hominis* (Frgm.).

Paris, Bibl. Nationale, Coislin., 332; s. XV.

Alexander Aphrodisiensis: (f. 1) *Quarundam difficultatum solutiones.*
Alexander Aphrodisiensis: (f. 32ᵛ) *Problematum physicorum et medicorum eclogae. Libr IV* (Capita 291).

Paris, Bibl. Nationale, Coislin., 334; s. XV.

Ioannes Zacharias Actuarius:
(f. 1) *De methodo medendi libri VI.*
(f. 19) *De methodo medendi libri VI.*
(f. 215) *De urinis libri VII.*

Paris, Bibl. Nationale, Coislin., 335; s. XV.

Antonius Pyropulus: (f. 1) *Excerpta* (Remedium pro tussi).
Cyrillus Alexandrinus: (f. 1) *Excerpta* (Formulae remediorum variae, inter quas ... Cyrilli Alexandr. fragmentum).
Rufus: (f. 8) *Excerpta varia* (De aquis. »*Aus* Orib.« Wellmann).
Diocles: (f. 10) *Ad Antigonum regem epistula de tuenda valetitudine.*
Paulus Aegineta: (f. 69) *De succedaneis, ex Galeno.*
Meletius monachus: (f. 75) *Iatrosophia/Excerpta varia* (Jatros. Gal. Hipp. et Melet. Cap. DCIV).

Paris, Bibl. Nationale, Coislin., 384; s. XIV.

Meletius monachus: (f. 162) *De natura hominis.*

Paris, Bibl. Nationale, Imprimés, Rés. Te 138.27; s. XV.

Dioscurides: (f. 44ᵛ) *De mensuris et ponderibus* (Frgm.).

Paris, Bibl. Nationale, Parisin.
Now Paris, Bibliothèque nationale de France, *graeci*

Paris, Bibl. Nationale, Parisin. 36; s. XIV–XV.

Paulus Aegineta: (f. 96) *Excerpta varia* (Pauli Aeg. Excerpta ex Hipp. et Gal. de venae sectione).
Dionysius Simplex: (f. 164v) *De fabrica hominis.*

Paris, Bibl. Nationale, Parisin. 396; s. XIII.

Diocles: (f. 455) *Ad Antigonum regem epistula de tuenda valetitudine.*
Herophilus Sophista: (f. 445) *De alimentis, quae singulis mensibus sumenda aut vitanda sunt.*

Paris, Bibl. Nationale, Parisin. 476; s. X.

Gregorius Nyssenus: (f. 64v) *De hominis opificio.*

Paris, Bibl. Nationale, Parisin. 478; s. XV.

S. Basilius: (f. 105v) *De hominis generatione. Libri III.*

Paris, Bibl. Nationale, Parisin. 479; s. XIII–XV.

Gregorius Nyssenus: (f. 79) *De hominis opificio.*

Paris, Bibl. Nationale, Parisin. 500; s. XI.

S. Basilius: (f. 184v) *De hominis generatione. Libri III.*

Paris, Bibl. Nationale, Parisin. 503; s. XIV.

Gregorius Nyssenus: (f. 144) *De hominis opificio.*

Paris, Bibl. Nationale, Parisin. 777 A; s. XVI.

Gregorius Nyssenus: (f. 246v) *De hominis opificio.*

Paris, Bibl. Nationale, Parisin. 825; s. XVI.

Nemesius Emesenus: (f. 1) *De natura hominis.*
Theophilus: (f. 108) *De hominis fabrica libri V.*

Paris, Bibl. Nationale, Parisin. 826; s. XVI.

Nemesius Emesenus: *De natura hominis.*

Paris, Bibl. Nationale, Parisin. 827; s. XVI.

Nemesius Emesenus: *De natura hominis.*

Paris, Bibl. Nationale, Parisin. 827 A; s. XVI.

Nemesius Emesenus: *De natura hominis* (Frgm. Nemesii? Inc. Τὴν κακίαν Πλωτῖνος μέν).

Paris, Bibl. Nationale, Parisin. 834; a. 1585.

Epiphanius: (f. 1) *Physiologus* (cum lat. versione et notis D. Consali Ponce de Leon Hispalensis).

Paris, Bibl. Nationale, Parisin. 835; s. XVI.

Epiphanius: (f. 206v) *De mensuris et ponderibus II.*

Paris, Bibl. Nationale, Parisin. 912; s. XIV.

Ioannes Chrysostomus: (f. 266) *De adversa valetudine et medicis.*
S. Basilius: (f. 519) *Ad Eusthatum medicum de obiectionum haereticorum solutione.*

Paris, Bibl. Nationale, Parisin. 940; s. XV.

Gregorius Nyssenus: (f. 140) *De hominis opificio.*

Paris, Bibl. Nationale, Parisin. 956; s. XIV.

Gregorius Nyssenus: (f. 82v) *De hominis opificio.*

Paris, Bibl. Nationale, Parisin. 968; s. XV.

Gregorius Nyssenus: (f. 109) *De hominis opificio.*

Paris, Bibl. Nationale, Parisin. 985; s. XV, XVI.

Stephanus Atheniensis: (f. 71) *De febrium differentiis ex ore Theophili.*
Herophilus Sophista: (f. 315v) *De alimentis, quae singulis mensibus sumenda aut vitanda sunt.*

Paris, Bibl. Nationale, Parisin. 993; s. XIV.

Theophylactus Simocatta: (f. 231v) *Quaestiones naturales.*

Paris, Bibl. Nationale, Parisin. 1000; s. XIV.

Ioannes Chumnos: (f. 156 [?]) *Quali victus ratione podagra evitari* (Sub nomine Nicephori Chumni?).

Paris, Bibl. Nationale, Parisin. 1007; s. X–XI.

Gregorius Nyssenus: (f. 1) *De hominis opificio.*

Paris, Bibl. Nationale, Parisin. 1009; s. XVI.

Gregorius Nyssenus: (f. 1) *De hominis opificio.*

Paris, Bibl. Nationale, Parisin. 1010; s. XVI.

Gregorius Nyssenus: (f. 105) *De hominis opificio.*
Symeon S. Mamas: (f. 175) *De mutationibus quae corpori et animae accidunt ex aëre, elementis et cibis.*

Paris, Bibl. Nationale, Parisin. 1044; s. XIV.

Nemesius Emesenus: (f. 1) *De natura hominis* (*beginnt c. 2, p. 102 I Matth., schließt 368, 10; abgeschr. aus Dresd. Da 57* [above p. 32]).

Paris, Bibl. Nationale, Parisin. 1045; a. 1501.

Nemesius Emesenus: (f. 1) *De natura hominis.*

Paris, Bibl. Nationale, Parisin. 1046; s. XVI.

Nemesius Emesenus: *De natura hominis.*

Paris, Bibl. Nationale, Parisin. 1053; s. X–XI.

Gregorius Nyssenus: (f. 207) *De hominis opificio.*

Paris, Bibl. Nationale, Parisin. 1247; s. XIV–XV.

Gregorius Nyssenus: (f. 52) *De hominis opificio.*

Paris, Bibl. Nationale, Parisin. 1268; s. XII.

Nemesius Emesenus:
(f. 53) *De natura hominis.*
(f. 295v) *Quarundam difficultatum solutiones.*

Paris, Bibl. Nationale, Parisin. 1277; s. XIII.

Gregorius Nyssenus: (f. 55) *De hominis opificio.*

Paris, Bibl. Nationale, Parisin. 1310; s. XV.

Splenius philosophus: (f. 443v) *De generatione hominis* (Sine auct. nomine).

Paris, Bibl. Nationale, Parisin. 1346; s. XI–XII.

Splenius philosophus: (f. 274) *De generatione hominis* (Sine auct. nomine).

Paris, Bibl. Nationale, Parisin. 1389; s. XVI.

Cyrillus Alexandrinus: (f. 387v) *De mensuris et ponderibus.*

Paris, Bibl. Nationale, Parisin. 1405; s. XVI.

Hermes Trismegistus: (f. 42) *Iatromathematica ad Ammonium Aegyptium.*

Paris, Bibl. Nationale, Parisin. 1542; s. X–XIII.

Gregorius Nyssenus: (f. 10) *De hominis opificio.*

Paris, Bibl. Nationale, Parisin. 1603; s. XVI.

Dioscurides: (f. 178) *Excerpta.*
Nemesius Emesenus: (f. 224) *De natura hominis.*

Paris, Bibl. Nationale, Parisin. 1630; s. XIV.

Theophilus:
De urinis.
(f. 22) *De alvi excrementis.*
Alexander Aphrodisiensis: (f. 181) *Quarundam difficultatum solutiones.*
Macarius Magnes: (f. 205) *De urinis.*
Menander iatrosophista: (f. 212v) *De mulieribus.*
Andromachus: (f. 217v) *Excerpta* (Remedia in podagram).

Paris, Bibl. Nationale, Parisin. 1631; s. XIV–XVI.

Diocles: (f. 168^{v}) *Ad Antigonum regem epistula de tuenda valetitudine.*

Paris, Bibl. Nationale, Parisin. 1739; s. XV.

Nemesius Emesenus: (f. 340) *De natura hominis.*

Paris, Bibl. Nationale, Parisin. 1766; s. XVII.

Splenius philosophus: (f. 437) *De generatione hominis* (Sine auct. nomine).

Paris, Bibl. Nationale, Parisin. 1788; a. 1440.

Splenius philosophus: (f. 238^{v}) *De generatione hominis* (Σπλ. φίλοσ. π. γενέσ. καὶ ὅθεν τρίτα καὶ ἔννατα καὶ τεσσαρακοστά).

Paris, Bibl. Nationale, Parisin. 1848; s. XV.

Alexander Aphrodisiensis: (f. 136) *De mixtione.*

Paris, Bibl. Nationale, Parisin. 1865; s. XV.

Alexander Aphrodisiensis: (f. 8^{v}) *Excerpta varia.*
Paulus Aegineta: (f. 133) *Excerpta varia.*

Paris, Bibl. Nationale, Parisin. 1868; s. XIV, XV.

Erotianus: *Vocum Hippocraticarum conlectio.*

Paris, Bibl. Nationale, Parisin. 1883; s. XIV.

Aëtius Amidenus: *Iatricorum libri XVI* (*Apogr. von Parisin. 2191* [p. 118]).
Oribasius:
Excerpta varia (*Vgl.* D.-Buss. I p. XXXVI).
Medicae collectiones ad Iulianum (L. III 65 [bis]. VII 26 [*vgl.* Oribas. II praef. p. 5 *und* p. 90 sq.]. cap. 26–40 libror. incert.).
Alexander Aphrodisiensis: (f. 1) *Problematum physicorum et medicorum eclogae. Libri V.*
Theophilus: (f. 74^{v}–156) *Commentarius in Hippocratis aphorismos* (Sine auctor. nomine. Inc. mutil. τεχνικῆς φάμεν. *Vgl.* Costomiris, Rev. des ét. gr. II [1889] p. 357).
Aëtius Amidenus: (f. 180^{v}) *Iatricorum libri XVI* (*Coll. mit der Ald. im Berol. fol. 39 [275]* [above p. 15]).

Paris, Bibl. Nationale, Parisin. 1884; a. 1503.

Alexander Aphrodisiensis: (f. 1) *Problematum physicorum et medicorum eclogae. Libri V.*
Gregorius Nyssenus: (f. 78) *De pulsibus* (Fragmentum).

Paris, Bibl. Nationale, Parisin. 1893; s. XVI.

Alexander Aphrodisiensis: (f. 153) *Problematum physicorum et medicorum eclogae. Libri V* (Libri II).

Paris, Bibl. Nationale, Parisin. 1943; s. XVI.

Cassius iatrosophistes: (f. 43^{v}) *Quaestiones medicae et problemata physica* (Quaestt. medicae de animalibus et quadrupediis).

Paris, Bibl. Nationale, Parisin. 1991; s. XV.

Hermes Trismegistus:
(f. 25) *Iatromathematica ad Ammonium Aegyptium.*
(f. 29^{v}) *Excerpta varia* (Exc. de rebus medico-astrologicis).
Pancharius, **Petosiris**, **Zenarius**: (f. 29^{v}) *Excerpta* (Excerpta de rebus medico-astrologicis).
Zenarius: (f. 49) *Exordia.*

Paris, Bibl. Nationale, Parisin. 2027; a. 1449.

Epiphanius: (f. 213) *Physiologus.*

Paris, Bibl. Nationale, Parisin. 2028; s. XV–XVI.

Alexander Aphrodisiensis: (f. 107) *De nutritione et augmento.*

Paris, Bibl. Nationale, Parisin. 2037; s. XVI.

Melampus:
(f. 41) *De palpitatione divinatio ad regem Ptolemaeum.*
(f. 54) *De naevis corporis.*

Paris, Bibl. Nationale, Parisin. 2047; s. XV.

Alexander Aphrodisiensis: (f. 6) *Problematum physicorum et medicorum eclogae. Libri V* (Frgm.).
Theophilus: (f. 16^{v}) *Excerpta varia* (Fragm. de phlebotomia).
Paulus Aegineta: (f. 30) *Epitomae medicae libri septem.*

Paris, Bibl. Nationale, Parisin. 2047 A; s. XIV.

Alexander Aphrodisiensis: (f. 1) *Problematum physicorum et medicorum eclogae. Libri* (Frgm. Libri II, initio mutili).
Cassius iatrosophistes: (p. 51) *Quaestiones medicae et problemata physica.*
Meletius monachus: (f. 113v) *De natura hominis.*

Paris, Bibl. Nationale, Parisin. 2048; s. XV.

Alexander Aphrodisiensis: (f. 1) *Problematum physicorum et medicorum eclogae. Libri V* (Libri II).

Paris, Bibl. Nationale, Parisin. 2077; s. XV.

Nemesius Emesenus: (f. 66) *De natura hominis.*

Paris, Bibl. Nationale, Parisin. 2098; s. XIII.

Ioannes Zacharias Actuarius: (f. 119) *De spiritu animali libri II.*

Paris, Bibl. Nationale, Parisin. 2118; s. XVI.

Melampus: (f. 56) *De palpitatione divinatio ad regem Ptolemaeum.*

Paris, Bibl. Nationale, Parisin. 2139; s. XVII.

Hermes Trismegistus: (f. 1) *Iatromathematica ad Ammonium Aegyptium.*
Pancharius: (f. 70v) *Compendium de decubitu infirmorum.*
Hermes Trismegistus: (f. 88) *Canon de decubitu infirmorum.*
Petosiris:
(f. 90) *De decubitu infirmorum.*
(f. 115) *Epistula ad regem Nechepso.*

Paris, Bibl. Nationale, Parisin. 2140; s. XII–XIII.

Soranus: (f. 8v) *Hippocratis genus et vita secundum Soranum.*

Paris, Bibl. Nationale, Parisin. 2141; s. XV.

Erotianus: *Vocum Hippocraticarum conlectio.*
Soranus: (f. 8) *Hippocratis genus et vita secundum Soranum.*

Paris, Bibl. Nationale, Parisin. 2142; s. XIII–XIV.

Erotianus: *Vocum Hippocraticarum conlectio.*
Soranus: (f. 12) *Hippocratis genus et vita secundum Soranum.*

Paris, Bibl. Nationale, Parisin. 2143; s. XIV.

Erotianus: *Vocum Hippocraticarum conlectio.*
Soranus: (f. 10) *Hippocratis genus et vita secundum Soranum.*

Paris, Bibl. Nationale, Parisin. 2144; s. XIV.

Erotianus: *Vocum Hippocraticarum conlectio.*
Ioannes Zacharias Actuarius: *Excerpta varia.*
Soranus: (f. 12) *Hippocratis genus et vita secundum Soranum.*

Paris, Bibl. Nationale, Parisin. 2145; s. XV.

Erotianus: *Vocum Hippocraticarum conlectio.*
Soranus: *Hippocratis genus et vita secundum Soranum.*

Paris, Bibl. Nationale, Parisin. 2147; s. XVI.

Stephanus Ἀρχιατρὸς τῶν Μαγγάνων: (f. 30) *Excerpta varia.*

Paris, Bibl. Nationale, Parisin. 2148; s. XV.

Erotianus: *Vocum Hippocraticarum conlectio.*

Paris, Bibl. Nationale, Parisin. 2149; s. XVI.

Theophilus: (f. 1–94^{v}) *Commentarius in Hippocratis aphorismos.*
Nicolaus Myrepsus: (f. 102) *De compositione medicamentorum, alphabetice* (»Desunt B–Z«).
Oribasius: (f. 159) *De ponderibus et mensuris* (De mensuris et ponderibus ex Orib. et Gal.)
Esdras Propheta: (f. 165^{v}) *De diebus criticis.*
Paulus Aegineta: (f. 177) *Epitomae medicae libri septem* (Lib. de fracturis).
Oribasius: (f. 201) *Excerpta varia* (Orib. et Gal. capita varia de re medica).

Paris, Bibl. Nationale, Parisin. 2150; a. 1584.

Damascius: *Expositio in aphorismos Hippocratis. Sectiones VII.*

Paris, Bibl. Nationale, Parisin. 2151; s. XVI.

Rufus:
(f. 1) *De corporis humani appellationibus.*
(f. 6–12) *Nomenclatura rerum ad hominem pertinentium. Libri III.*
Oribasius: (f. 12) *Medicae collectiones ad Iulianum* (L. XXIV. XXV).

Erotianus: (f. 49) *Vocum Hippocraticarum conlectio* (A-O).
Dioscurides: (f. 65) *Liber agens de experientia medica, de simplicibus et compositis medicamentis, ordine literarum digestus* (*Wie im* cod. Bibl. Io. Rhodii [above p. 100]).
Stephanus Atheniensis: (f. 65) *Dioscoridis et Stephani Atheniensis de pharmacis ordine literarum.*

Paris, Bibl. Nationale, Parisin. 2152; s. 1539.

Muscio: (f. 1) *De morbis mulierum.*
Rufus: (f. 6) *Excerpta varia* (Frgm. de rebus venereis. » *Aus* Orib.« Wellmann).

Paris, Bibl. Nationale, Parisin. 2153; XV.

Aëtius Amidenus: (f. 218–289) *Excerpta varia* (*Vgl.* Rose, Soranus p. 412 ss).
Soranus: (f. 220) *De muliebribus affectionibus* (*Vgl.* Buss.-Dbg. Oribasius I p. xxv).
Ioannes Zacharias Actuarius:
(f. 290) *De methodo medendi libri VI* (L. I–V).
(f. 408) *De urinis libri VII.*
Paulus Aegineta: (f. 424v) *De succedaneis, ex Galeno.*
Ioannes Zacharias Actuarius: (f. 435) *De spiritu animali libri II.*
Paulus Aegineta:
(f. 435) *Excerpta varia* (De spiritu animali, ad Josephum rhacendytam).
(f. 447) *Excerpta varia* (De diaeta, ad Josephum rhacendytam).
(f. 458) *De urinis.*

Paris, Bibl. Nationale, Parisin. 2154; s. XIV.

Melampus: (f. 280) *De palpitationibus* (*De palpitatione divinatio ad regem Ptolemaeum*).

Paris, Bibl. Nationale, Parisin. 2155; s. XIV.

Theophilus: (f. 1v, 265) *De hominis fabrica libri V.*
Gregorius Nyssenus: (f. 305) *Oratio adversus astronomos* (Frgm.).

Paris, Bibl. Nationale, Parisin. 2177; s. XVI.

Oribasius: (f. 10) *Ad Eunapium de parabilibus medicamentis. Libri IV.*
Erotianus: (f. 96) *Vocum Hippocraticarum conlectio.*

Paris, Bibl. Nationale, Parisin. 2178; s. XIV, XV.

Theophilus: (f. 1) *Excerpta varia* (Excerpta de pulsibus).
Paulus Aegineta: *Excerpta varia*:
(f. 9) *De praenotionibus.*
(f. 11v) *De febrium differentiis.*
Alexander Trallianus: *Excerpta varia:*
(f. 11v) *De febrium differentiis.*
(f. 42) *De morbis hominum et remediis.*
Paulus Aegineta: (f. 44) *Excerpta varia* (De morbis hominum et remediis).

Paris, Bibl. Nationale, Parisin. 2179; s. IX.

Dioscurides: *De materia medica* (Lib. II [101] 202 – V 124).

Paris, Bibl. Nationale, Parisin. 2180; s. XV.

Dioscurides: (f. 1) *De materia medica* (Frgm.).
Hermes Trismegistus:
(f. 85v) *Ad Asclepium de plantis XII zodiaci signorum.*
(f. 85v) *Ad Asclepium de plantis VII planetarum* (Frgm.).

Paris, Bibl. Nationale, Parisin. 2181; s. XVI.

Dioscurides: (f. 1) *Liber agens de experientia medica, de simplicibus et compositis medicamentis, ordine literarum digestus* (*Wie im* cod. Bibl. Io. Rhodii [above p. 101]).
Stephanus Atheniensis: (f. 1) *Dioscoridis et Stephani Atheniensis de pharmacis ordine literarum.*

Paris, Bibl. Nationale, Parisin. 2182; a. 1481.

Dioscurides:
(f. 7) *De materia medica.*
(f. 134 *und* 148) *Metaphrasis in Nicandri Theriaca et Alexipharmaca.*
(f. [148 s] 134) *De iis, quae virus eiaculantur, animalibus libellus, in quo et de rabioso cane.*
(f. 174v) *De venenis eorumque praecautione et medicatione.*

Paris, Bibl. Nationale, Parisin. 2183; s. XV.

Crateuas: *De herbis* (Frgm. Codex Dioscuridis interpolati).
Dioscurides: (f. 1) *De materia medica.*
Porphyrius: (f. 7) *Excerpta.*

Dioscurides:
(f. 147) *De venenis eorumque praecautione et medicatione.*
(f. 147 *und* 155) *Metaphrasis in Nicandri Theriaca et Alexipharmaca.*
(f. 154) *De iis, quae virus eiaculantur, animalibus libellus, in quo et de rabioso cane.*
(f. 163^{v}) *Opera varia* (Notha).

Paris, Bibl. Nationale, Parisin. 2184; s. XVI.

Dioscurides:
(f. 1) *De materia medica* (alphab.).
(f. 188) *De venenis eorumque praecautione et medicatione.*
(f. 188 *und* 197) *Metaphrasis in Nicandri Theriaca et Alexipharmaca.*
(f. 197^{v}) *De iis, quae virus eiaculantur, animalibus libellus, in quo et de rabioso cane.*
Theophilus: (f. 221^{v}) *De pulsibus.*

Paris, Bibl. Nationale, Parisin. 2185; s. XVI.

Dioscurides:
(f. 1) *De materia medica.*
(f. 175) *De venenis eorumque praecautione et medicatione.*
(f. 175 *und* 184) *Metaphrasis in Nicandri Theriaca et Alexipharmaca.*
(f. 184) *De iis, quae virus eiaculantur, animalibus libellus, in quo et de rabioso cane.*
(f. 194^{v}) *Opera varia* (Notha).

Paris, Bibl. Nationale, Parisin. 2186; s. XVI.

Aretaeus:
(f. 1) *De causis et signis acutorum morborum libri II.*
(f. 1) *De causis et signis diuturnorum morborum libri II.*
(f. 50^{v}) *De curatione acutorum morborum libri II.*
(f. 50^{v}) *De curatione diuturnorum morborum libri II.*

Paris, Bibl. Nationale, Parisin. 2187; s. XVI.

Aretaeus:
(f. 1^{v}) *De causis et signis acutorum morborum libri II.*
(f. 1^{v}) *De causis et signis diuturnorum morborum libri II.*
(f. 68) *De curatione acutorum morborum libri II.*
(f. 68) *De curatione diuturnorum morborum libri II.*

Paris, Bibl. Nationale, Parisin. 2188; s. XV.

Oribasius: (f. 1) *Conspectus ad Eustathium filium. Libri II.*

Paris, Bibl. Nationale, Parisin. 2189; s. XVI.

Oribasius: *Medicae collectiones ad Iulianum* (Libri XV).

Paris, Bibl. Nationale, Parisin. 2190; s. XV.

Oribasius: *Medicae collectiones ad Iulianum* (Libri I–X).

Paris, Bibl. Nationale, Parisin. 2191; s. XIV.

Aëtius Amidenus: (f. 1) *Iatricorum libri XVI* (*Coll. mit der Ald. im Berol. fol. 39 [275]* [above p. 15]).
Africanus: (f. 344) *De ponderibus et mensuris.*
Paulus Aegineta: (f. 435) *Epitomae medicae libri septem* (L. VI usque ad c. 120 χειρισμόν).

Paris, Bibl. Nationale, Parisin. 2192; s. XV.

Aëtius Amidenus: (f. 3) *Iatricorum libri XVI* (*Apogr. von [Parisin.] 2191* [above]).
Africanus: (f. 316v) *De ponderibus et mensuris* (*Abschrift von [Parisin.] 2191; vgl.* Costomiris Rev. des ét. gr. III [1890] 167).
Paulus Aegineta: (f. 317v) *Epitomae medicae libri septem* (L. VI 8–122).

Paris, Bibl. Nationale, Parisin. 2193; s. XIV, XV.

Aëtius Amidenus: (f. 1) *Iatricorum libri XVI.*
Rufus: (f. 400–401) *Conspectus de pulsibus* (Sonst dem Galen zugeschriebenes Werk).
Africanus: (f. 402) *De ponderibus et mensuris.*

Paris, Bibl. Nationale, Parisin. 2194; x. XV.

Aëtius Amidenus: (f. 3) *Iatricorum libri XVI* (L. V–XIV).
Constantinus Meliteniota: (f. 400v) *De antidotis libri II.*
Euphemius Siculus, Philippus Xerus: (f. 454) *Medicamentorum compositiones ab Euph. S. et Philippo Nero Rheginensi collectae* (Βιβλίον περιέχον συνθέσεις συναχθὲν καὶ πειραθὲν παρὰ Εὐφημίου Σικελοῦ τοῦ θαυμασιωτάτου καὶ Φιλίππου Ξηροῦ τοῦ Ῥιγινοῦ τῶν θαυμασίων ἰατρῶν. Inc. Σύνθεσιν σὺν θεῷ τροχίσκον) [Treu]).

Paris, Bibl. Nationale, Parisin. 2195; s. XIII.

Aëtius Amidenus: (f. 1) *Iatricorum libri XVI* (L. V–VIII).

Paris, Bibl. Nationale, Parisin. 2196; s. XI.

Aëtius Amidenus: *Iatricorum libri XVI* (L. IX–XII; L. IX–XII 49 μαλάγματα διάφορα).

Paris, Bibl. Nationale, Parisin. 2197; s. XVI.

Aëtius Amidenus: *Iatricorum libri XVI* (L. XIII–XVI).

Paris, Bibl. Nationale, Parisin. 2198; a. 1522.

Aëtius Amidenus: (f. 1) *Iatricorum libri XVI.*

Paris, Bibl. Nationale, Parisin. 2199; s. XVI.

Aëtius Amidenus: *Iatricorum libri XVI* (L. V. VI 1–55. IX–XV).

Paris, Bibl. Nationale, Parisin. 2200; s. XV.

Alexander Trallianus: (f. 1) *Therapeutica. Libri XII.*

Paris, Bibl. Nationale, Parisin. 2201; s. XV.

Alexander Trallianus: (f. 1) *Therapeutica. Libri XII.*

Paris, Bibl. Nationale, Parisin. 2202; s. XVI.

Alexander Trallianus: (f. 1) *Therapeutica. Libri XII.*
Aretaeus:
(f. 141) *De curatione diuturnorum morborum libri II* (init. et fine mutil.).
(f. 147) *De causis et signis acutorum morborum libri II.*
(f. 154v) *De causis et signis diuturnorum morborum libri II.*
(f. 175v) *De curatione acutorum morborum libri II.*

Paris, Bibl. Nationale, Parisin. 2203; s. XVI.

Alexander Trallianus: *Therapeutica. Libri XII* (L. I et II fine mutil.).

Paris, Bibl. Nationale, Parisin. 2204; s. XVI.

Alexander Trallianus: (f. 7) *Therapeutica. Libri XII* (fine mutil.).
Theophilus: (f. 23) *De urinis.*

Paulus Aegineta: (f. 43) *Epitomae medicae libri septem* (Liber VI).

Paris, Bibl. Nationale, Parisin. 2205; s. XI.

Paulus Aegineta: *Epitomae medicae libri septem* (Libri VII, fine mutili).

Paris, Bibl. Nationale, Parisin. 2206; s. XI.

Paulus Aegineta: *Epitomae medicae libri septem* (Libri VII, fine mutil.).

Paris, Bibl. Nationale, Parisin. 2207; a. 1299 (1294).

Paulus Aegineta: (f. 1) *Epitomae medicae libri septem.*

Paris, Bibl. Nationale, Parisin. 2208; s. XI–XV, XIV.

Paulus Aegineta: (f. 1) *Epitomae medicae libri septem.*
Oribasius: (f. 285^{v}) *Excerpta varia* (Opuscula).
Adamantius, Oribasius: (f. 385) *Excerpta* (Oribasii et Adamantii fragmenta de ponderibus et mensuris. *Gedruckt* Orib. V 85).

Paris, Bibl. Nationale, Parisin. 2209; s. XVI.

Paulus Aegineta: (f. 1) *Epitomae medicae libri septem* (Libri VII, fine mutil.).

Paris, Bibl. Nationale, Parisin. 2210; a. 1357 (1537).

Paulus Aegineta: (f. 1) *Epitomae medicae libri septem.*
Damnastes: (f. 368) *Excerpta.*
Iacobus Psychrestus: (f. 368) *Excerpta.*
Palladius: (f. 368) *Excerpta varia.*

Paris, Bibl. Nationale, Parisin. 2211; s. XVI.

Paulus Aegineta: *Epitomae medicae libri septem.*

Paris, Bibl. Nationale, Parisin. 2212; s. XV.

Paulus Aegineta: *Epitomae medicae libri septem* (Libri VII, fine mutil.).

Paris, Bibl. Nationale, Parisin. 2213; s. XVI.

Paulus Aegineta: *Epitomae medicae libri septem.*

Paris, Bibl. Nationale, Parisin. 2214; s. XVI.

Paulus Aegineta: *Epitomae medicae libri septem.*

Paris, Bibl. Nationale, Parisin. 2215; s. XVI.

Paulus Aegineta: *Epitomae medicae libri septem* (Libri VII, fine mutil.).

Paris, Bibl. Nationale, Parisin. 2216; s. XVI–XI.

Paulus Aegineta: *Epitomae medicae libri septem* (L. I–III, fine mutil.).

Paris, Bibl. Nationale, Parisin. 2217; s. XI–XV.

Paulus Aegineta: (f. 1) *Epitomae medicae libri septem* (L. III 28 – VII).
Adamantius: (f. 285ᵛ) *Excerpta.*

Paris, Bibl. Nationale, Parisin. 2218; s. XVI.

Palladius: (f. 1) *Stephani philosophi vel Palladii synopsis de febribus.*
Stephanus Atheniensis: (f. 1) *De febrium differentiis ex ore Theophili* (Stephanus [vel Palladii] synopsis de febribus).

Paris, Bibl. Nationale, Parisin. 2219; s. XV.

Theophilus: (f. 1) *De pulsibus.*

Paris, Bibl. Nationale, Parisin. 2220; s. XVI.

Aretaeus: *De causis et signis acutorum morborum libri II.*
Stephanus Alexandrinus: *In Magni sophistae librum de urinis* (Στεφάνου σχόλαια μάγνου εἰς τὸ περὶ οὔρων).
Theophilus: (f. 1) *De urinis.*
Stephanus Magnes: (f. 24ᵛ) *Scholia in (Theophili?) tractatum de urinis.*
Theophilus: (f. 28) *De pulsibus.*
Rufus: (f. 44) *De corporis humani appellationibus.*
Aretaeus: (f. 76) *De curatione acutorum morborum libri II* (L. I).

Paris, Bibl. Nationale, Parisin. 2222; s. XV.

Stephanus Atheniensis: *In aphorismos Hippocratis commentarius* (sub nomine Meletii).
Theophilus: *Commentarius in Hippocratis aphorismos* (Sub nomine Meletii).
Meletius monachus: (f. 104) *In aphorismos Hippocratis commentarius.*

Paris, Bibl. Nationale, Parisin. 2223; s. XVI.

Stephanus Atheniensis: *In aphorismos Hippocratis commentarius* (Apogr. *von* nr. [Parisin.] 2222 [above]).
Theophilus: *Commentarius in Hippocratis aphorismos* (*Apograph. von* [Parisin.] 2222).
Meletius monachus: (f. 158) *In aphorismos Hippocratis commentarius.*

Paris, Bibl. Nationale, Parisin. 2224; s. XIV ex., XIV–XV, XV.

Meletius monachus: (f. 1) *De natura hominis* (Libri II).
Nicomedes Iatrosophista: (f. 71) *Lexicon.*
Photius monachus: (f. 76) *Carmina* (Carmina de terra, oceano, nubilus et sanguine).
Ioannes Archiatrus: (f. 80) *Variorum morborum curatio* (»Opus medicum«).
Dioscurides:
(f. 284) *De materia medica* (Libri VIII).
(f. 427ᵛ) *De venenis eorumque praecautione et medicatione.*
(f. 434ᵛ) *De iis, quae virus eiaculantur, animalibus libellus, in quo et de rabioso cane.*

Paris, Bibl. Nationale, Parisin. 2225; s. XIV.

Meletius monachus: (f. 1) *De natura hominis.*
Nemesius Emesenus: (f. 50) *De natura hominis.*

Paris, Bibl. Nationale, Parisin. 2226; XVI.

Meletius monachus: *De natura hominis.*

Paris, Bibl. Nationale, Parisin. 2227; s. XVI.

Meletius monachus: *De natura hominis.*

Paris, Bibl. Nationale, Parisin. 2228; s. XI, XII, XIV–XV.

Epiphanius: (f. 49) *De duodecim gemmis panno sacerdotis infibulatis.*
Orpheus: (f. 50) *De lapidibus.*
Stephanus Atheniensis: (f. 55) *De febrium differentiis ex ore Theophili* (Stephani synopsis de variis febrium generibus).
Severus: (f. 57ᵛ) *De instrumentis infusoriis seu clysteribus ad Timotheum* (de intestinis).
Theophilus: (f. 59) *Excerpta varia* (Exc. de excrementis).

Philagrius: (f. 63) *Excerpta varia* (Opusculum de urinis, ex Galeno, Philagrio etc.).
Dioscurides: (f. 92) *Excerpta*.
Theophilus: (f. 95–149^{v}) *Commentarius in Hippocratis aphorismos*.
Aëtius Amidenus: (f. 150) *Iatricorum libri XVI* (L. V. VI praeter capp. 97 dimid. et 98. VII. VIII partim. X).

Paris, Bibl. Nationale, Parisin. 2229; s. XIII, XIV.

Stephanus Alexandrinus: *In Magni sophistae librum de urinis* (Σχόλια Στεφάνου μάγνου εἰς τὸ περὶ οὔρων).
Diocles: (f. 25) *Hippocratis vel, ut alii volunt, Dioclis epistula ad Ptolemaeum Aegypti regem*.
Theophilus: (f. 35^{v}) *De urinis*.
Stephanus Magnes: (f. 42) *Scholia in (Theophili?) tractatum de urinis*.
Theophilus: (f. 46^{v}) *De pulsibus*.

Paris, Bibl. Nationale, Parisin. 2230; s. XIV.

Alexander Aphrodisiensis: (f. 123^{v}) *Problematum physicorum et medicorum eclogae. Libri V* (Problemata physica 150).
Aëtius Amidenus: *Iatricorum libri XVI*:
(f. 156) L. V.
(f. 195) L. VIII.

Paris, Bibl. Nationale, Parisin. 2232; s. XV.

Ioannes Zacharias Actuarius:
(f. 1) *De urinis libri VII* (L. I. II., ceterorum frgmta.).
(f. 63) *De spiritu animali libri II*.

Paris, Bibl. Nationale, Parisin. 2233; s. XVI.

Ioannes Zacharias Actuarius: *De methodo medendi libri VI* (L. I–V et index l. VI).

Paris, Bibl. Nationale, Parisin. 2234; s. XVI.

Ioannes Zacharias Actuarius: *De spiritu animali libri II*.

Paris, Bibl. Nationale, Parisin. 2235; s. XVI.

Ioannes Zacharias Actuarius: *De methodo medendi libri VI*:
(f. 1) De medicamentorum compositione liber V.

(f. 88) De ratione medendi Liber IV.

Paris, Bibl. Nationale, Parisin. 2236; s. XV.

Ioannes Archiatrus: (f. 1) *Variorum morborum curatio* (»Hoc opus ab Omont Actuario adscriptum Daremberg Not. et Extr. I 23 Ioanni Archiatro attribuit«).
Ioannes Zacharias Actuarius: (f. 1) *In Galenum de methodo medendi* (Capp. 152).
Gregorius Theologus: (f. 59^{v}) *Alatium*.

Paris, Bibl. Nationale, Parisin. 2237; s. XIV.

Oribasius: *Medicae collectiones ad Iulianum* (L. IX 52–55. X 13. 14. 19–36. XXI. XXII. LIV. XXIV 30–36. c. 21 librorum incert. XXI 7 bis).
Nicolaus Myrepsus: (f. 7) *De compositione medicamentorum, alphabetice*.
Aëtius Amidenus: (f. 163) *Iatricorum libri XVI* (Frgm. L. IV–X).
Oribasius, Aëtius Amidenus: (f. 165^{v}) *Excerpta varia* (Collectionis medicinalis ex Galeno Orib. Aetio libri IV–X).

Paris, Bibl. Nationale, Parisin. 2238; s. XV.

Nicolaus Myrepsus: (f. 1) *De compositione medicamentorum, alphabetice*.
Dioscurides: (f. 539) *Liber agens de experientia medica, de simplicibus et compositis medicamentis, ordine literarum digestus*.

Nationale, Bibl. Nationale, Parisin. 2240; s. XVI.

Chariton: (f. 1) *De pastillis, pillulis, zulapiis et clysteribus*.
Paulus Aegineta: (f. 40) *De succedaneis, ex Galeno*.
Oribasius: *Excerpta varia*:
(f. 45) De antidotis, emplastris, oleis.
(f. 92^{v}) De plantis et metallis.
Rufus: (f. 146^{v}) *Excerpta varia* (Gal. et Rufi excerpta de venereis »Aus Orib.« Wellmann).
Meletius monachus: (f. 151^{v}) *Excerpta varia* (Versus politici de urinis illarumque differentiis).
Mnesitheus Cyzicenus: (f. 156) *Excerpta* (Fragmentum de brassica. Inc. Κράμβην χρὴ κατακόψαι [Aus Oribas. I 278 sq.]).
Alexander: (f. 156^{v}) *Hippocratis vel Alexandri epistula ad Ptolemaeum regem*.

Paris, Bibl. Nationale, Parisin. 2243; a. 1339.

Nicolaus Myrepsus: (f. 11v) *De compositione medicamentorum, alphabetice.*
Dioscurides: (f. 553) *Liber agens de experientia medica, de simplicibus et compositis medicamentis, ordine literarum digestus.*
Oribasius: (f. 640) *Excerpta varia* (De mensuris et ponderibus).
Hermes Trismegistus:
(f. 654v) *Ad Asclepium de plantis XII zodiaci signorum* (Anonym.).
Ad Asclepium de plantis VII planetarum (Anonym.).

Paris, Bibl. Nationale, Parisin. 2244; s. XIV–XV.

Lampudes: (f. 95v) (Ἐκ τὸ χορτηνὸν [sic !] τοῦ Λαμπούδη).
Diocles: (f. 253v) *Ad Antigonum regem epistula de tuenda valetitudine.*

Paris, Bibl. Nationale, Parisin. 2247; s. XVI.

Apollonius Citiensis: *Commentarius in Hippocratis de articulis, libri III.*
Erotianus: *Vocum Hippocraticarum conlectio.*
Oribasius: *Medicae collectiones ad Iulianum* (L. XLVI–XLIX).
Rufus: *De corporis humani appellationibus* (*Apographon des* [Flor.] Laurent. [plut. 74, 7] [above p. 42]).

Paris, Bibl. Nationale, Parisin. 2248; s. XVI.

Apollonius Citiensis: *Commentarius in Hippocratis de articulis, libri III.*
Erotianus: *Vocum Hippocraticarum conlectio.*
Oribasius: *Medicae collectiones ad Iulianum* (*Wie im* Parisin. 2247 [above]).
Rufus: *De corporis humani appellationibus* (*Apographon des* [Flor.] Laurent. [plut. 74, 7] [above p. 42]).

Paris, Bibl. Nationale, Parisin. 2249; s. XVI.

Zosimus Panopolita:
(f. 1) *Liber de virtute et compositione aquarum.*
(f. 18) *De sacra divinaque arte auri et argenti faciendi.*
(f. 94v) *De instrumentis et fornacibus.*
(f. 96) *Gemini commentarii de aqua divina* (II).

Paris, Bibl. Nationale, Parisin. 2251; s. XVII.

Zosimus Panopolita: (f. 145) *De sacra divinaque arte auri et argenti faciendi.*

Paris, Bibl. Nationale, Parisin. 2252; s. XVII.

Zosimus Panopolita:
(f. 265) *Liber de virtute et compositione aquarum.*
(f. 219) *Gemini commentarii de aqua divina* (II).

Paris, Bibl. Nationale, Parisin. 2254; s. XV.

Erotianus: *Vocum Hippocraticarum conlectio.*

Paris, Bibl. Nationale, Parisin. 2255; s. XV.

Erotianus: *Vocum Hippocraticarum conlectio.*
Soranus: (f. 53^{v}) *Hippocratis genus et vita secundum Soranum.*

Paris, Bibl. Nationale, Parisin. 2256; s. XIV, XV.

Hermes Trismegistus: *Kyranides.*
Aëtius Amidenus: (f. 34) *Excerpta varia* (Synopsis simplic. Gal. medicamentorum; libri II. *Vgl.* den Scorial. Σ. III. 17 [above p. 35]).
Ioannes Zacharias Actuarius:
(f. 144^{v}) *De urinis libri VII.*
(f. 240) *De spiritu animali libri II.*
(f. 280) *De methodo medendi Libri VI.*
Neophytus Prodromenus: (f. 540) *Remediorum collectio alphabetica.*
Hermes Trismegistus:
(f. 580) *Ad Asclepium de plantis VII planetarum.*
(f. 584^{v}) *De decanis ad Asclepium.*
(f. 588^{v}) *Ad Asclepium de plantis VII planetarum.*

Paris, Bibl. Nationale, Parisin. 2257; s. XVI.

Meletius monachus: (f. 239) *De natura hominis.*
Theophilus:
(f. 345) *De urinis.*
(f. 363^{v}) *De pulsibus.*

Paris, Bibl. Nationale, Parisin. 2260; s. XVI.

Magnus Emesenus: (f. 9) *De urinis.*
Ioannes Zacharias Actuarius:
(f. 42) *Tractatus de urinis, qui ex Avicenna translatus dicitur in graecam linguam a Christodulo, in ordinem redactus ab Actuario Zacharia.*
(f. 42–120) *De urinis libri VII.*

Stephanus Magnes: (f. 98–120) *Scholia in (Theophili?) tractatum de urinis.*
Stephanus Alexandrinus: (f. 178ᵛ) *In Magni sophistae librum de urinis* (Inscr. *wie im* [Cheltenham] Phillipps. 6763 [above p. 31]).
Dioscurides: (f. 260) *De materia medica* (Libri IV fine mutil.).

Paris, Bibl. Nationale, Parisin. 2261; s. XVI.

Rufus: (f. 1) *Nomenclatura rerum ad hominem pertinentium. Libri III.*
Oribasius: (f. 37) *Medicae collectiones ad Iulianum* (L. XXIV–XLIX).

Paris, Bibl. Nationale, Parisin. 2262; s. XVI.

Rufus: (f. 1) *Nomenclatura rerum ad hominem pertinentium. Libri III.*
Oribasius: (f. 31) *Medicae collectiones ad Iulianum* (*Wie im* Parisin. 2261).

Paris, Bibl. Nationale, Parisin. 2263; s. XVI.

Rufus: (f. 1) *Nomenclatura rerum ad hominem pertinentium. Libri III.*
Oribasius: (f. 28ᵛ) *Medicae collectiones ad Iulianum* (*Wie im* Parisin. 2261 [above]).

Paris, Bibl. Nationale, Parisin. 2264; s. XVI.

Rufus: *De corporis humani appellationibus* (fine mutil.).

Paris, Bibl. Nationale, Parisin. 2267; s. XIV, XV.

Stephanus Atheniensis: (f. 55ᵛ) *De febrium differentiis ex ore Theophili.*

Paris, Bibl. Nationale, Parisin. 2269; s. XV.

Palladius: (f. 84) *Stephani philosophi vel Palladii synopsis de febribus.*

Paris, Bibl. Nationale, Parisin. 2270; s. XV–XVI.

Aëtius Amidenus: (f. 177) *Iatricorum libri XVI* (L. XVI inscr. Γαλ. περὶ γυναικειων παθῶν).
Ioannes Zacharias Actuarius: (f. 231) *De urinis libri VII.*

Paris, Bibl. Nationale, Parisin. 2275; a. 1465.

Cleopatra: (f. 1) *De mensuris et ponderibus.*
Democritus: (f. 7ᵛ) *Physica et mystica.*
Synesius: (f. 14) *Ad Dioscorum, scholia in librum Democriti* (§§ 1–5).

Paris, Bibl. Nationale, Parisin. 2276; s. XVI.

Stephanus Atheniensis: (f. 191) *De febrium differentiis ex ore Theophili.*
Archigenes, Philagrius: (f. 217) *Excerpta varia* (Archigenis et Philagrii opusculum de renum calculis, ex Aëtio).

Paris, Bibl. Nationale, Parisin. 2286; s. XIV.

Neophytus Prodromenus: *Remediorum collectio alphabetica.*
Dioscurides: (f. 1) *Liber agens de experientia medica, de simplicibus et compositis medicamentis, ordine literarum digestus.*
Crateuas: (f. 1–54v) *De herbis* (Frgm. Excerpta continentur opere Dioscuridis περὶ ῥιζῶν κτλ.).
Olymnius Alexandrinus: (f. 55) *Excerpta* (Excerpta de criticis diebus etc.).
Archigenes, Asclepiades, Diocles, Timocrates: (f. 89) *Excerpta* (Remedia ad sedandos dentium dolores).
Neophytus Prodromenus: (f. 105. 108v) *Remediorum collectio alphabetica.*
Ioannes Episcopus Prisdianensis: (f. 114) *Collectanea de urinis* (Inscr. Περὶ οὔρων διάγνωσις καὶ πραγματεία ἀρίστη. Inc. Τὴν περὶ τῆς τῶν οὔρων διαφορᾶς πραγματείαν. [Treu]).
Theophilus: (f. 121v) *Excerpta varia* (Περὶ χρωμάτων).
Dioscurides: (f. 124) *Excerpta* (Praecepta de sanitate tuenda per XII menses).
Ioannes Episcopus Prisdianensis:
(f. 127v) *Collectanea de intestinis, ex Palladio, Archelao, Stephano Alexandrino etc.*
(f. 136) *Collectanea de excrementis* (Expl. τοὺς ἐν βάθει πάσχοντας ἀφανεῖν τόπους. [Treu]).

Paris, Bibl. Nationale, Parisin. 2287; s. XV–XVI.

Dioscurides: (f. 1) *De materia medica* (Libri VI fine mutil.).

Paris, Bibl. Nationale, Parisin. 2288; s. XVI.

Aretaeus:
(f. 1) *De causis et signis acutorum morborum libri II.*
(f. 1) *De causis et signis diuturnorum morborum libri II.*
(f. 89) *De curatione acutorum morborum libri II.*
(f. 89) *De curatione diuturnorum morborum libri II* (in fine mut.).
Rufus: (f. 161) *De vesicae renumque affectibus.*

Paris, Bibl. Nationale, Parisin. 2289; s. XVI.

Aretaeus:
(f. 1) *De causis et signis acutorum morborum libri II.*
(f. 1) *De causis et signis diuturnorum morborum libri II.*
(f. 88) *De curatione acutorum morborum libri II.*

Paris, Bibl. Nationale, Parisin. 2290; s. XVIII.

Xenocrates: (f. 1) *De alimento ex aquatilibus.*

Paris, Bibl. Nationale, Parisin. 2291; s. XVI.

Xenocrates: *De alimento ex aquatilibus.*

Paris, Bibl. Nationale, Parisin. 2292; s. XIV.

Paulus Aegineta: *Epitomae medicae libri septem.*

Paris, Bibl. Nationale, Parisin. 2293; s. XIV.

Paulus Aegineta: *Epitomae medicae libri septem* (L. I–III, initio et fine mutili, graece et arabice).

Paris, Bibl. Nationale, Parisin. 2294; s. XV.

Paulus Aegineta:
(f. 1) *Epitomae medicae libri septem* (Frgm. L. VII 3).
(f. 73^v) *Excerpta varia* (Collectio remediorum).
(f. 124) *Excerpta varia* (Exc. medica).
Dioscurides: (f. 138) *Excerpta* (De plantis et animalibus Exc.).

Paris, Bibl. Nationale, Parisin. 2295; s. XIV.

Palladius: *Scholia in Hippocratis de popularibus morbis librum sextum, sectiones VIII.*
Nemesius Emesenus: (f. 50) *De natura hominis.*

Paris, Bibl. Nationale, Parisin. 2296; s. XVI.

Theophilus: (f. 1–131^v) *Commentarius in Hippocratis aphorismos.*
Stephanus Alexandrinus: (f. 131^v–277^v), *Scholia in Hippocratis praenotiones. Sectiones III* (*Vgl.* Costomiris, Rev. des ét. gr. II [1889] p. 356).

Paris, Bibl. Nationale, Parisin. 2297; s. XVI.

Theophilus: *De hominis fabrica libri V.*

Paris, Bibl. Nationale, Parisin. 2298; s. XVI.

Stephanus Magnes: *Empirica.*

Paris, Bibl. Nationale, Parisin. 2299; s. XV.

Meletius monachus:
(f. 1) *De natura hominis.*
(f. 89v) *De anima.*
(f. 99v) *De quattuor elementis.*
Nemesius Emesenus: (f. 104) *De natura hominis.*
S. Basilius: (f. 191) *De hominis generatione. Libri III.*

Paris, Bibl. Nationale, Parisin. 2300; a. 1569.

Meletius monachus: *De natura hominis.*

Paris, Bibl. Nationale, Parisin. 2301; s. XII–XIV.

Diocles: (f. 124) *Hippocratis vel, ut alii volunt, Dioclis epistula ad Ptolemaeum Aegypti regem.*

Paris, Bibl. Nationale, Parisin. 2304; s. XV.
See also **Oxford, Bibl. Bodl., Baroccian 2304** above (p. 96).

Ioannes Zacharias Actuarius:
(f. 1) *De urinis libri VII.*
(f. 114) *De spiritu animali libri II.*
(f. 191) *De methodo medendi Libri VI.*

Paris, Bibl. Nationale, Parisin. 2305; a. 1418.

Ioannes Zacharias Actuarius:
(f. 1) *De urinis libri VII.*
(f. 121) *De spiritu animali libri II.*
(f. 158) *De methodo medendi Libri VI.*

Paris, Bibl. Nationale, Parisin. 2306; s. XV.

Ioannes Zacharias Actuarius:
(f. 1) *De urinis libri VII.*

(f. 289) *De spiritu animali libri II.*
Theophilus:
(f. 329) *De urinis.*
(f. 338) *De alvi excrementis.*

Paris, Bibl. Nationale, Parisin. 2307; s. XVI.

Ioannes Zacharias Actuarius:
Tractatus de urinis, qui ex Avicenna translatus dicitur in graecam linguam a Christodulo, in ordinem redactus ab Actuario Zacharia.
(f. 1) *De urinis libri VII.*
(f. 122–451v) *De methodo medendi Libri VI.*
(f. 453v) *De spiritu animali libri II.*
Theophilus:
(f. 508v) *De urinis.*
(f. 523v) *De alvi excrementis.*
Mercurius monachus: (f. 599) *De pulsibus.*

Paris, Bibl. Nationale, Parisin. 2308; s. XV.

Theophilus: (f. 27) *De urinis.*
Ioannes Zacharias Actuarius:
(f. 55) *De urinis libri VII* (ab init. mutil.).
(f. 204v) *De spiritu animali libri II.*

Paris, Bibl. Nationale, Parisin. 2313; s. XIV.

Dioscurides: (f. 1) *Excerpta* (Remedia varia).
Paulus Aegineta: (f. 1) *Excerpta varia* (Remedia varia).

Paris, Bibl. Nationale, Parisin. 2314; s. XIV–XV.

Herophilus Sophista: (f. 87) *De alimentis, quae singulis mensibus sumenda aut vitanda sunt.*
Andreas Caesareae in Cappadocia Archiepiscopus: (f. 345v) *Interrogationes et responsiones ex libro II. Therapeuticae.*

Paris, Bibl. Nationale, Parisin. 2315; s. XV.

Mercurius monachus: (f. 1) *De pulsibus* (»Περὶ σφυγμῶν κάλλιστον καλλίστου ἀνδρὸς μοναχοῦ μερκουρίου. Inc. Τὸ σῶμα τοῦ ἀνθρώπου. Expl. κατὰ τὴν ἡμετέραν δύναμιν ἐξεθέμεθα« Treu.).
Meletius monachus: (f. 11v) *Excerpta varia* (*Wie im* Parisin. 2240 [above p. 124]).

Paulus Aegineta: (f. 64^{v}) *De succedaneis liber* (Pauli Aeginetae frgm. ex Galeno de succ.).
Ioannes Antiochenus Archiatrus: (f. 117) *Collectio remediorum ex Dioscoride, Hippocrate et Galeno.*
Nicolaus Myrepsus: (f. 276) *De emplastris.* »... muß fort Parisin. 2315; f. 276. Da steht nur ἑρμενία νικολάου, περὶ ἐμπλάστρου πάνυ ὠφέλιμον ...« Treu.

Paris, Bibl. Nationale, Parisin. 2316; s. XV.

Ioannes Iatrosophista: (f. 51^{v}) *De morbis eorumque curationibus.*
Theophilus: (f. 170) *De urinis.*
Mangens (?): (f. 191) *De urinis, De urinis compendium* (Galeni et Mangentis synopsis de urinis).
Gregorius Nyssenus: (f. 194) *De pulsibus.*
Alexander (Trallianus ?): (f. 207^{v}) *Opusculum de pulsuum dignotione in febricitantibus et aphorismi de urinis.*
Paulus Aegineta: (f. 229^{v}) *Excerpta varia.*

Paris, Bibl. Nationale, Parisin. 2318; s. XV.

Paulus Aegineta: (f. 72) *De succedaneis, ex Galeno.*

Paris, Bibl. Nationale, Parisin. 2320; s. XVI.

Paulus Aegineta: (f. 12^{v}) *Excerpta varia* (Π. φλεβοτομίας).
Athenaeus: (f. 18^{v}) *Synopsis de urinis* (Expl. εἰς θάνατον ὤποια [sic !]).
Cleopatra: (f. 216^{v}) *De mensuris et ponderibus.*

Paris, Bibl. Nationale, Parisin. 2321; s. XVI.

Rufus: (f. 1) *De corporis humani appellationibus* (Sine auctoris nomine. Inc. Περὶ ὀφθαλμοῦ. Τῶν δὲ τοῦ ὀφθαλμοῦ).
Oribasius: (f. 11^{v}) *Medicae collectiones ad Iulianum* (*Wie im* Parisin. 2261 [above p. 127]).

Paris, Bibl. Nationale, Parisin. 2324; s. XVI.

Erasistratus, **Magnus Emesenus**: (f. 1) *Iatrosophia* (Hippocratis, Galeni, Magni et Erasistrati iatrosophium. Inc. Τὴν περὶ τῆς τῶν οὔρων).
Herodotus: (f. 146^{v}–209^{v}) *Diagnostica de morbis acutis et chronicis* (Inc. Τῶν σκοτωματικῶν τὴν αἰτίαν = Parisin. Suppl. 636 [see below p. 140]. f. 46^{v}).

Paris, Bibl. Nationale, Parisin. 2325; s. XIII.

Democritus: (f. 8ᵛ) *Physica et mystica.*
Synesius: (f. 20) *Ad Dioscorum, scholia in librum Democriti.*
Zosimus Panopolita:
(f. 86. 82) *Gemini commentarii de aqua divina* (I. II).
(f. 118) *De sacra divinaque arte auri et argenti faciendi.*

Paris, Bibl. Nationale, Parisin. 2326; s. XVI.

Democritus: (f. 1) *Physica et mystica.*

Paris, Bibl. Nationale, Parisin. 2327; a. 1478.

Cleopatra: (f. 15) *De mensuris et ponderibus.*
Democritus: (f. 24ᵛ) *Physica et mystica.*
Synesius: (f. 72ᵛ) *Ad Dioscorum, scholia in librum Democriti.*
Zosimus Panopolita:
(f. 80. 83) *Gemini commentarii de aqua divina* (ll. I–II).
(f. 85) *Liber de virtute et compositione aquarum.*
(f. 112) *De sacra divinaque arte auri et argenti faciendi.*
(f. 220) *Gemini commentarii de aqua divina* (ll. I–II).
Democritus: (f. 258) *Liber V ad Leucippum.*
Hermes Trismegistus: (f. 293) *Organum.*

Paris, Bibl. Nationale, Parisin. 2329; s. XVI–XVII.

Zosimus Panopolita:
(f. 41) *De sacra divinaque arte auri et argenti faciendi.*
(f. 183ᵛ) *Gemini commentarii de aqua divina* (I).

Paris, Bibl. Nationale, Parisin. 2331; s. XVII.

Rufus:
(f. 1) *De medicamentis purgantibus.*
(f. 11ᵛ) *De vesicae renumque affectibus.*

Paris, Bibl. Nationale, Parisin. 2334; s. XVI.

Aretaeus:
(f. 1) *De causis et signis acutorum morborum libri II.*
(f. 1) *De causis et signis diuturnorum morborum libri II.*
(f. 219) *De curatione acutorum morborum libri II.*
(f. 219) *De curatione diuturnorum morborum libri II.*

Paris, Bibl. Nationale, Parisin. 2335; s. XVI.

Oribasius: *Ad Eunapium de parabilibus medicamentis. Libri IV.*

Paris, Bibl. Nationale, Parisin. 2336; s. XVI.

Ioannes Spensatus: *Liber de incurabilibus et difficile curabilibus morbis.*

Paris, Bibl. Nationale, Parisin. 2337; s. XV–XVI.

Oribasius: (f. 1) *Excerpta varia* (Anon. collectio medicorum, ex Oribasio etc.).
Paulus Aegineta: (f. 11) *Excerpta varia* (De fracturis etc.).
Dioscurides: (f. 89) *Excerpta* (Exc. De simplicibus remediis).

Paris, Bibl. Nationale, Parisin. 2381; s. XV.

Adamantius: (f. 80^{v}) *De ventis.*
Alexander Aphrodisiensis: (f. 93) *Problematum physicorum et medicorum eclogae. Libri V* (Problemata physica).

Paris, Bibl. Nationale, Parisin. 2408; s. XIII.

Marcellus Sidetes: (f. 216^{v}) *Medicina ex piscibus.*
Oribasius: (f. 224^{v}) *Excerpta varia* (S. Artemii martyris, Iuliani imp. et Oribasii medici dialogus de Apolline Delphico).

Paris, Bibl. Nationale, Parisin. 2419; ca, a. 1460, s. XV.

Hermes Trismegistus: *Kyranides.*
Orpheus: *De lapidibus.*
Hermes Trismegistus: (f. 265^{v}) *Ad Asclepium de plantis XII zodiaci signorum.*

Paris, Bibl. Nationale, Parisin. 2422; s. XVI.

Timotheus Gazaeus: *De animalibus quadrupedis physicisque eorum facultatibus.*

Paris, Bibl. Nationale, Parisin. 2426; s. XVI.

Petosiris: (f. 6^{v}) *Organum de vita et morte.*
Hermes Trismegistus, Petosiris, Protagoras, Pythagoras: (f. 16^{v}) *Iatromathematica ad Ammonium Aegyptium* (Frgm. *Protagorae [Pythagorae] excerpta ex iatromathematicis Mercurii et Petosiridis etc. astrologica.*
Epiphanius: (f. 90) *Physiologus.*

Paris, Bibl. Nationale, Parisin. 2428; s. XVI.

Nemesius Emesenus: (f. 116) *De natura hominis* (Sub nomine Adamantionis).

Paris, Bibl. Nationale, Parisin. 2502; s. XVI.

Hermes Trismegistus:
Kyranides (Lib. III. II. IV).
(f. 1) *Ad Asclepium de plantis XII zodiacui signorum.*
(f. 19) *De decanis ad Asclepium.*
(f. 30v) *Ad Asclepium de animalium proprietatibus et remediis quae ex illis peti possunt.*

Paris, Bibl. Nationale, Parisin. 2506; s. XIII.

Hermes Trismegistus: *De XII locorum nomenclatura et facultate.*

Paris, Bibl. Nationale, Parisin. 2509; s. XV.

Epiphanius: (f. 188) *Physiologus.*

Paris, Bibl. Nationale, Parisin. 2510; a. 1384, s. XIV.
Possibly also **[Paris, B. R. 349]** above (p. 102).

Oribasius: *Medicae collectiones ad Iulianum* (L. I 5. 15–65. II 1–53. III. 21 26–28. 31–34 abbrev.).
Dioscurides: (f. 80) *De animalibus marinis et terrestribus ad morbos curandos idoneis.*
Paulus Aegineta, **Theophilus**: (f. 108) *Excerpta varia* (Pracepta medica et remedia varia).
Oribasius: (f. 125) *Excerpta varia* (Remedia varia, inter quae ... Oribasii).
Lucas: (f. 125) *Excerpta varia* (Remedia varia, inter quae S. Lucae etc.).

Paris, Bibl. Nationale, Parisin. 2537; a. 1272.

Hermes Trismegistus: *Kyranides.*
Kyranus: *Opus physico-magicum de naturalibus virtutibus.*

Paris, Bibl. Nationale, Parisin. 2540; s. XVI.

Alexander Aphrodisiensis: (f. 93) *De mixtione.*

Paris, Bibl. Nationale, Parisin. 2596; s. XIV.

Soranus: (f. 184) *Hippocratis genus et vita secundum Soranum.*

Paris, Bibl. Nationale, Parisin. 2614; s. XVI.

Erotianus: *Vocum Hippocraticarum conlectio.*

Paris, Bibl. Nationale, Parisin. 2615; s. 1533 *und* 1584.

Erotianus: *Vocum Hippocraticarum conlectio.*
Macarius Maximus: (f. 9) *De anima.*

Paris, Bibl. Nationale, Parisin. 2633; s. XIII.

Marcellus Sidetes: (f. 743) *Medicina ex piscibus* (fine mutil.).

Paris, Bibl. Nationale, Parisin. 2651; s. XVI.

Erotianus: (f. 1) *Vocum Hippocraticarum conlectio.*

Paris, Bibl. Nationale, Parisin. 2665; s. XIV–XV.

Epiphanius:
(f. 204) *De mensuris et ponderibus.*
(f. 204–210) *De mensuris et ponderibus I.*

[Paris, Bibl. Nationale, Parisin. 2671 (?); s. XV].

Theophilus: *Commentarius in Hippocratis Aphorismos.*

Paris, Bibl. Nationale, Parisin. 2720; s. XVI.

Africanus: (f. 186v) *De ponderibus et mensuris.*
Epiphanius: (f. 186v) *De mensuris et ponderibus.*

Paris, Bibl. Nationale, Parisin. 2726; s. XV.

Aglaias: *Ad suffusiones Aglaiae ..., Alexandri discipuli, condiscipuli Demosthenis et amici, versus heroelegi.*

Paris, Bibl. Nationale, Parisin. 2731; s. XVI.

Africanus: (f. 133v) *De ponderibus et mensuris.*
Epiphanius: (f. 133v) *De mensuris et ponderibus.*

Paris, Bibl. Nationale, Parisin. 2830; a. 1515.

Africanus: (f. 232) *De ponderibus et mensuris.*
Epiphanius: (f. 232) *De mensuris et ponderibus.*

Paris, Bibl. Nationale, Parisin. 2847; s. XVI.

Diocles: (f. 137) *Ad Antigonum regem epistula de tuenda valetitudine.*
Aëtius Amidenus: (f. 139) *Excerpta varia.*

Paris, Bibl. Nationale, Parisin. 2894; s. XIII, XV–XVI.

Libanius: (f. 336) *De hominis generatione.*
Splenius philosophus: (f. 336) *De generatione hominis* (Sub nomine Libanii).

Paris, Bibl. Nationale, Parisin. 3023; s. XV–XVI.

Splenius philosophus: (f. 46v) *De generatione hominis* (Sine autor. nomine).

Paris, Bibl. Nationale, Parisin. 3044; s. XV.

Alexander Aphrodisiensis: (f. 69) *Problematum physicorum et medicorum eclogae. Libri V* (Problemata).

Paris, Bibl. Nationale, Parisin. 3076; a. 1616.

Archigenes: (f. 56) *Excerpta* (De nephritide).
Oribasius: (f. 56) *Excerpta varia* (De nephritide).

Paris, Bibl. Nationale, Parisin. 3099; s. –.

Oribasius: (f. 13) *Conspectus ad Eustathium filium. Libri IX* (Frgm.).

Paris, Bibl. Nationale, Suppl.
Now Paris, Bibliothèque nationale de France, supplément grec

Paris, Bibl. Nationale, Suppl. 3; a. 1616.

Dioscurides: *Excerpta* (Thesaurus Theophrasti et D. auctore Paulo Renealmo Blesensi).

Paris, Bibl. Nationale, Suppl. 49; s. XVI.

Meletius monachus: (f. 1) *De natura hominis.*

Paris, Bibl. Nationale, Suppl. 64; s. XV–XVII.

Theophilus: (f. 207–230v) *Commentarius in Hippocratis aphorismos* (Sine auctor. nomine. Expl. λειποθυμία καὶ συγκοπὴ ἕπεται. *Vgl.* Costomiris l. l. p. 357).

Paris, Bibl. Nationale, Suppl. 84; s. XVI.

Meletius monachus: *De natura hominis.*

Paris, Bibl. Nationale, Suppl. 86; s. XVII.

Nemesius Emesenus: *De natura hominis.*

Paris, Bibl. Nationale, Suppl. 148; s XVI.

Nemesius Emesenus: *De natura hominis.*

Paris, Bibl. Nationale, Suppl. 165; s. XV.

Alexander Sophista: (f. 116) *De hominis generatione.*

Paris, Bibl. Nationale, Suppl. 194; s. XVI.

Nemesius Emesenus: (f. 2) *De natura hominis* (Sub nomine Adamantii).

Paris, Bibl. Nationale, Suppl. 270; s. XVII.

Apollonius Citiensis: (f. 351) *Commentarius in Hippocratis de articulis, libri III.*

Paris, Bibl. Nationale, Suppl. 338; s. XIV.

Paulus Aegineta: (f. 1) *Epitomae medicae libri septem.*

Paris, Bibl. Nationale, Suppl. 341; a. 1533–1535.

Gregorius Nyssenus: (f. 10) *De hominis opificio.*

Paris, Bibl. Nationale, Suppl. 445; s. XIX.

Opp. c. mss. bibl. reg. a M. Myna collata.
Aretaeus:
De causis et signis acutorum morborum libri II.
De curatione acutorum morborum libri II.
De causis et signis diuturnorum morborum libri II.
De curatione diuturnorum morborum libri II.

Paris, Bibl. Nationale, Suppl. 446; s. X.

Oribasius:
Medicae collectiones ad Iulianum (Frgm. L. XLIV 5–8. 23. XLV 26 *und* Ἐκλογαὶ βοηθημάτων).

(f. 35ᵛ–38ᵛ) *Excerpta varia* (Ὀφθαλμικά; *vgl.* Costomiris Revue des ét. gr. III [1890] 148).

Petosiris: (f. 43) *Epistula ad regem Nechepso* (Inc. Ψῆφος σεληνιακός).

Stephanus Atheniensis: (f. 107) *De febrium differentiis ex ore Theophili.*

Paulus Aegineta: (f. 114) *Epitomae medicae libri septem* (L. VI 1–63 omissis capp. 15–21).

Leo: (f. 147–168) *Synopsosis artis medicae.*

Oribasius: (f. 168) *Excerpta varia* (Eclogae ex Orib. *Vgl.* Dbg.-Buss. I p. XXXVI. Littré, Revue de philologie II [1846–47]).

Paris, Bibl. Nationale, Suppl. 493; s. XIX.

Dioscurides:

De materia medica (Variae lectt. e codice Athoo Βιβλ. μον. Λαύρας [Ω 75] [above p. 11] a Myna collato).

Excerpta (Variae lectt. in D.).

Paris, Bibl. Nationale, Suppl. 494; s. XV.

Paulus Aegineta: (f. 5) *Epitomae medicae libri septem.*

Paris, Bibl. Nationale, Suppl. 629; s. XIX.

Theophilus:

(f. 1) *De urinis.*

(f. 9ᵛ) *De alvi excrementis.*

(f. 33) *Excerpta varia* (Variae lectiones in Theophilum, e cod. Parisin. 2220 [above p. 121]).

Stephanus Magnes: (f. 43) *Scholia in (Theophili?) tractatum de urinis.*

Theophilus: (f. 45) *De pulsibus.*

Rufus: (f. 72) *De corporis humani appellationibus.*

Soranus: (f. 91) *De matrice et muliebri pudendo.*

Lycus: (f. 94ᵛ) *De vulva et muliebri pudendo* (*Wohl aus* Oribas. III p. 382).

Paris, Bibl. Nationale, Suppl. 630–632; s. XIV, XI, XIX.

Aëtius Amidenus: *Iatricorum libri XVI* (L. I. VI–XII. XIII–XVI).

Paris, Bibl. Nationale, Suppl. 633; s. XIX.

Aretaeus: *De causis et signis acutorum morborum libri II* (Var. lectt. e codd. Paris. 2186. 2187. [above p. 117] 2202. [above p. 119] 2220. [above p. 121] 2288. 2289. [above p. 129] 2334 [above p. 133]).

Paris, Bibl. Nationale, Suppl. 636; s. XVI.

Herodotus: (f. 21–82) *Diagnostica de morbis acutis et chronicis* (Expl. καὶ ὑπὸ τῆς διαπύρου. *Vgl.* Costomiris, Rev. des ét. gr. III [1890] p. 146).
Esdras Propheta: (f. 134) *De diebus criticis.*

Paris, Bibl. Nationale, Suppl. 637; s. XV.

Meletius monachus: (f. 7) *De natura hominis.*
Theophilus:
(f. 40) *De alvi excrementis.*
(f. 44) *De urinis.*
Ioannes Episcopus Prisdianensis: (f. 50) *Collectanea de urinis.*
Rufus: (f. 65v) *Quaestiones medicinales.*
Aëtius Amidenus: (f. 67v) *Excerpta varia* (De cephalalgia).

Paris, Bibl. Nationale, Suppl. 638; s. XV.

Ioannes Dioecetas Constantinopolitanus: (f. 1) *De medicina* (Libri VI–X).

Paris, Bibl. Nationale, Suppl. 639; s. XVIII.

Vincentius Damodes: *Physiologia.*

Paris, Bibl. Nationale, Suppl. 640; s. XVI.

Nemesius Emesenus: *De natura hominis.*

Paris, Bibl. Nationale, Suppl. 641; s. XVIII.

Nemesius Emesenus: *De natura hominis.*

Paris, Bibl. Nationale, Suppl. 652; s. XV.

Hermes Trismegistus: (f. 291) *Iatromathematica ad Ammonium Aegyptium.*

Paris, Bibl. Nationale, Suppl. 654; s. XIX.

Methodus Causocalybitus: (f. 224v) *De diaeta hominis.*

Paris, Bibl. Nationale, Suppl. 662; s. XIV.

Marcellus Sidetes: (f. 257v) *Medicina ex piscibus.*

Paris, Bibl. Nationale, Suppl. 682; s. X–XIX, XI.

Damascius: (f. 85) *Expositio in aphorismos Hippocratis. Sectiones VII* (Apogr. codicis [Parisin.] 2150 [above p. 114]).

Paris, Bibl. Nationale, Suppl. 683; s. XV–XVIII, XVIII.

Aëtius Amidenus: (f. 1ᵛ) *Excerpta varia* (Frgm.).
Oribasius: (f. 1ᵛ) *Excerpta varia*.
Aëtius Amidenus: (f. 55ᵛ) *Excerpta varia* (De symptomatibus urinarum).
Magnus Emesenus: (f. 58ᵛ) *De urinis* (»De urinarum differentiis«).

Paris, Bibl. Nationale, Suppl. 688; s. XVI.

Soranus: (f. 39) *Hippocratis genus et vita secundum Soranum*.

Paris, Bibl. Nationale, Suppl. 702; s. XV–XVI.

Nemesius Emesenus: (f. 43ᵛ) *De natura hominis*.

Paris, Bibl. Nationale, Suppl. 755; s. XIX.

Cornelius Celsus: (f. 123) *Fragmentum*.

Paris, Bibl. Nationale, Suppl. 764; s. XIV.

Alexander Trallianus: (f. 12) *Therapeutica. Libri XII* (Frgm. ex libro XI. sine auctoris nomine. Inscr. Εἰδήσεις ἰατρικαὶ διάφοροι).

Paris, Bibl. Nationale, Suppl. 836; s. XVII.

Alexander Aphrodisiensis: (f. 91) *De febribus*.

Paris, Bibl. Nationale, Suppl. 924; s. XV–XVI.

Paulus Aegineta: (f. 1) *Excerpta varia* (De differentia et causa aegritudinum).

Paris, Bibl. Nationale, Suppl. 1022; s. XVII.

Synesius: *Ad Dioscorum, scholia in librum Democriti*.
Democritus: (f. 1) *Physica et mystica*.

Paris, Bibl. Nationale, Suppl. 1098; s. XVI.

Dioscurides: *De materia medica* (Aldina a. 1518 cum collatt. et nott. mss. Angelii Vergetii et Ranconeti).

Paris, Bibl. Nationale, Suppl. 1156; s. IX–XI.
s. X.

Paulus Aegineta: (f. 23, 24, 25) *Epitomae medicae libri septem* (L. V–VI; = ed. Ald. fol. 77ᵛ l. 26 – fol. 78ᵛ l. 9; fol. 87ᵛ l. 11 – fol. 88 l. 13; fol. 95ᵛ l. 12 – fol. 96ʳ l. 13).

Paris, Bibl. Nationale, Suppl. 1193; s. XVI.

Paulus Aegineta: (f. 17) *De succedaneis, ex Galeno.*

Paris, Bibl. Nationale, Suppl. 1197; s. XI.
Possibly same as *graecus* **1297** below (*Census*: 261, nr [1394]).

Dioscurides: (f. 120) *De materia medica* (Frgm. libri IV).

Paris, Bibl. Nationale, Suppl. 1202; s. XIII, XIII–XVI, XIV–XVI.

Archigenes, **Dioscurides**, **Magnus Emesenus**, **Oribasius**, **Paulus Aegineta**, **Porphyrius**, **Socrates**: (f. 16) *Excerpta varia.*

Paris, Bibl. Nationale, Suppl. 1240; s. XI.

Aëtius Amidenus: *Iatricorum libri XVI* (L. I–VI a fine mutil. *Coll. im Berol. 39 [275]* [above p. 15]).

Paris, Bibl. Nationale, Suppl. 1297; s. XI.

Alexander Trallianus: (f. 1) *Therapeutica. Libri XII* (Frgm. *Vorlage des* [Venet.] Marcian. 295 [below p. 171]).
Paulus Aegineta: (f. 119ᵛ) *De mensuris et ponderibus.*
Soranus: (f. 127ᵛ) *De ponderibus et mensuris.*

Parma

Parma, Bibl. Palatina, Fondo De-Rossiano, 7; s. XV.
Now Ms. Parm. 3062 (*Census*: 262, nr [1399]).

Diocles: (f. 245) *Ad Antigonum regem epistula de tuenda valetitudine.*

Patmos

Patmos, Bibl. Monast. St. Ioann. Evang., –; s. X.
Possibly 202 (*Census*: 262, nr [1400]).

Nemesius Emesenus: *De natura hominis.*

Patmos, Bibl. Monast. St. Ioann. Evang., 11 (*bei* Coxe, Mss. gr. of the Levant); s. X.
Possibly 202 (*Census*: 263, nr [1402]).

Nemesius Emesenus: *De natura hominis* (*vgl.* nr. Λ' *bei* Migne, Patrol. gr. 149, 1049).

Patmos, Bibl. Monast. St. Ioann. Evang., 71 *bei* Coxe, Ms Gr of the Levant; s. XIII.
Possibly 208 (*Census*: 263, nr [1403]).

Paulus Aegineta: *Epitomae medicae libri septem* (»imperf.«).

Patmos, Bibl. Monast. St. Ioann. Evang., ΚΓ'.
Possibly 27 or 47 (*Census*: 263, nr [1404]).

Gregorius Nyssenus: *De hominis opificio* (*bei* Migne, Patrol. gr. 149 p. 1049).

Patmos, Bibl. Monast. St. Ioann. Evang., 111; s. –.
Possibly 208 (*Census*: 264, nr [1405]).

Paulus Aegineta: *Epitomae medicae libri septem* (»paraît fort ancien«).

Patmos, Bibl. Monast. St. Ioann. Evang., 277; s. XVII.

Aëtius Amidenus: *Iatricorum libri XVI* (L. IV).

Raudnitz

Raudnitz, –, 11; s. –.
Now Nelahozeves, Lobkowiczká, VI Fc 37 (*Census*: 266, nr [1410]).
Same as **VI F C 37** below.

Aëtius Amidenus: *Iatricorum libri XVI.*

Raudnitz, Bibl. Ducis Lobcovic, VI F C 37; s. XIV–XV.
Now Nelahozeves, Lobkowiczká, VI Fc 37 (*Census*: 266, nr [1411]).
See **11** above.

Aëtius Amidenus: *Iatricorum libri XVI* (L. VIII–XIV).

Rom, Bibl. Angelica
Roma, Biblioteca Angelica

Rom, Bibl. Angelica, 4 (C 4.16); s. XVI in.
Now Ang. gr. 4 (*Census*: 270, nr [1418]).

Paulus Nicaeensis: (f. 165) *De cognitione et curatione variorum morborum.*
Lucas: (f. 277ᵛ) *Compositio salsi intinctus.*
Esdras Propheta: (f. 290) *Pro hydropicis et omnibus morbis frigidis.*
Logadius: (f. 290) *Excerpta* (Σκευασία τῆς ἱερᾶς. Inc. Εἰς ξανθο⟨χο⟩λικούς, μελαγχολικούς, φλεγματικούς; N.56: εἰς ξανθοχολ. *usw. gehört zur Überschrift*).
Antonius Pyropulus: (f. 294) *Excerpta varia* (Ἑρμηνία).

Rom, Bibl. Angelica, 17 (C.5. 4); s. XIV.
Now Ang. gr. 17 (*Census*: 270, nr [1419]).

Ioannes Archiatrus: (f. 1) *Variorum morborum curatio* (Λόγοι καὶ ποίημα ἰωάννου ἀρχιατροῦ περιέχων συνοπτικὸς παντοίων παθῶν ἀδήλων καὶ φανερῶν τὴν θεραπείαν. Inc. Πρὸς πόνων κεφαλῆς. Κισσὸν ξήρανον εἰς ἥλιον. »Cf. Hardt III 212«).
Oribasius: (f. 91) *Excerpta varia* (Βίβλος περιέχουσα περὶ ἁπλῶν φαρμάκων, κράσεων καὶ μίξεων ὑγιεινῶν νοσούντων καὶ κτηνῶν ὁμοῦ καὶ τῶν πτηνῶν τῆς ἄγρας κτλ. Inc. Ἀπείρου σκευασία ξυροῦ. *Vgl.* [Oxford, Bodl.] Baroccian. 150. f. 20ᵛ [above p. 94]).
Meletius monachus:
(f. 141) *Excerpta varia* (Ἕτερα περὶ τροφῶν δυνάμεων ἐκβληθέντα ἐκ τῆς βίβλου τοῦ μοναχοῦ κυρίου Μελετίου · ἐκ τὸν μικρὸν [sic !] κόσμων).
(f. 141–236) *Excerpta varia* (Περὶ ἄρτου κατὰ ἀλφαβήτου. Inc. Τῶν ἄρτων ὅσοί ῥυπαροί. Expl. πρὸς ἀνθρωπίνου σώματος ὁμοιότητα).
Paulus Aegineta:
(f. 236) *Epitomae medicae libri septem* (Frgm. L. III 49).
(f. 238–238ᵛ) *Excerpta varia.*
Theophilus: (f. 247) *De urinis* (lacunos. et fine mutil.).

Philo: (f. 318) *Excerpta* (Ἀντίδοτος ἡ τοῦ Φίλωνος. Τοῖς ὑσακοληтικοῖς, πλευριτικοῖς καὶ πρὸς πᾶσαν ὀδύνην τὴν ἐντὸς κτλ. Expl. διάκλυζε καὶ στύονται · σκευάζεται δὲ ...).
Lucas: (f. 326) *Compositio salsi intinctus.*
Hermes Trismegistus: (f. 339) *Iatromathematica ad Ammonium Aegyptium* (Inc. mutil. καὶ ῥωννύντα = Idel. I p. 388, 8).

Rom, Bibl. Angelica, 68 (C.2.7); s. XV.
Now Ang. gr. 68 (*Census*: 270, nr [1420]).

Paulus Aegineta: *De succedaneis, ex Galeno.*

Rom, Bibl. Barberin.
Now at Città del Vaticano, Biblioteca Apostolica Vaticana, *Barberiniani*

Rom, Bibl. Barberin., I 17; s. XV.
Now *Vaticanus Barberinianus graecus* 17 (*Census*: 272, nr [1424]).

Democritus: (f. 13ᵛ) *De sympathicis et antipathicis.*

Rom, Bibl. Barberin., I 49; s. XV.
Now *Vaticanus Barberinianus graecus* 49 (*Census*: 272, nr [1425]).
See also **I 49 (= 359)** below.

Aëtius Amidenus: (f. 1–165) *Excerpta varia.*

Rom, Bibl. Barberin., I 49 (= 359); s. XVI.
Same as **I 49** above.
= *Vaticanus Barberinianus graecus* 49 (*Census*: 272, nr [1426]).

Soranus: (f. 1–165) *De muliebribus affectionibus* (Apogr. des Parisin. [2153] [above p. 115]).

Rom, Bibl. Barberin., I 72 (440); s. XVI.
Now *Vaticanus Barberinianus graecus* 72 (*Census*: 272, nr [1427]).

Perzoe: (f. 1) *Liber physiologicus ex India translatus et Chosroe regi Persarum traditus a Perzoe etc.*

Rom, Bibl. Barberin., I 91 (382); s. XV.
Now *Vaticanus Barberinianus graecus* 91 (*Census*: 272, nr [1429]).
See also **382 (I 91)** below (p. 147).

Rufus: (f. 1) *De medicamentis purgantibus* (Μονόβιβλον τίνας δεῖ καιθαίρειν καὶ ποίοις καθαρτηρίοις καί πότε. Inc. Οὔτε πάντας. Expl. στήθους καὶ πνεύματος).

Rom, Bibl. Barberin., I 118; s. IV, XIV, XV.
Now *Vaticanus Barberinianus graecus* 118 (*Census*: 273, nr [1430]).

Oribasius: (f. 1) *Conspectus ad Eustathium filium. Libri II.*
Dioscurides: (f. 293) *De mensuris et ponderibus* (Expl. τὸ ἐρυθρὸν τοῦ ξανθοῦ).

Rom, Bibl. Barberin., I 127; s. XVI.
Now *Vaticanus Barberinianus graecus* 127 (*Census*: 273, nr [1431]).

Proclus: *Excerpta* (Ἡ Πρόκλου ποδαγρικὴ καὶ πρὸς ἰσχιάδας).
Pancharius: (f. 197ᵛ) *Compendium de decubitu infirmorum.*
Antyllus: (f. 205ᵛ) *Excerpta* (Περὶ ἑψήσεως τῶν ἐμβαλλομένων εἰς τὰς ἐμπλάστρους φαρμάκων. Inc. Λιθαργυρ ... ἐν ταῖς ἕψησι. Expl. καταχέονται τὰ τηκτά).
Paulus Aegineta: (f. 206ᵛ) *Excerpta varia* (Περὶ τῶν ἀπὸ τῶν γευστῶν ποιοτήτων δηλουμένων κράσεων. Inc. Οὔτε ἐξ ὀσμῆς. Expl. καὶ στυπτηρία).
Alexander Rex: (f. 249ᵛ) *De septem herbarum facultate.*
Paulus Aegineta: (f. 252) *Excerpta varia* (Ὀδόντων προφυλακτικά. Inc. Οἱ ὀδόντες οὐκ. Expl. γλώττης φλέβας).
Maximus (Planudes?): (f. 261ᵛ) *De sanguinibus.*
Theophilus:
(f. 265) *De urinis* (Frgm. Inc. λευκὸν ὡς ὕδωρ. Expl. τὰ ἐλαιώδη καὶ δυσώδη).
f. 271) *De alvi excrementis* (Expl. τῷ συνετῷ δυνάμενον).
Paulus Aegineta: (f. 276) *Excerpta varia* (Πρὸς τεθλασμένους ὄνυχας, πρὸς ὑφαίμους ὄνυχας etc.).
Diocles: (f. 310) *Hippocratis vel, ut alii volunt, Dioclis epistula ad Ptolemaeum Aegypti regem.*
Paulus Aegineta:
(f. 311) *Excerpta varia* (Π. ἰχθύων Inc. Ὅτι μὲν πᾶς ἰχθύς. Expl. ὕδωρ ὁμοίως).
(f. 323) *Excerpta varia* (Π. ἑρμαφροδίτων. Inc. Τὸ ἑρμαφρόδιτον πάθος. Expl. θεραπευομένων).
(f. 334ᵛ) *Excerpta varia* (Ἡδυχρόου τοῦ ἐν τῇ θηριακῇ σκευασία).

Rom, Bibl. Barberin., II 58; s. XVI.
Now *Vaticanus Barberinianus graecus* 237 (*Census*: 273, nr [1433]).

Marianus: (f. 1) *Excerpta* (Εὑρισκόμενα ἐν ταῖς οὐσίαις Μαριάνου θουκκίου ἰατροῦ).

Dioscurides: (f. 47) *De iis, quae virus eiaculantur, animalibus libellus, in quo et de rabioso cane* (D. liber VII. Expl. ἰατρῶν σωθέντας ἔγνωμεν).

Rom, Bibl. Barberin., III 63 (= 245); s. XVI.
Now *Vaticanus Barberinianus graecus* 344 (*Census*: 273, nr [1434]).

Leo: (f. 376) *De hominis proprietatibus.*
Meletius monachus: (f. 394–414^{v}) *Jatrosophium* (Ἰατροσόφιον ἐκλελεγμένον Γαλ. Ἱππ. καὶ Μελετίου περὶ γυναικός. Expl. εἰς τὰ νευροχαλαστικά).

Rom, Bibl. Barberin., V 18; s. XI.
Now *Vaticanus Barberinianus graecus* 522 (*Census*: 273, nr [1435]).

Nemesius Emesenus: (f. 136^{v}) *De natura hominis* (Frgm.).

Rom, Bibl. Barberin., VI 5; s. XIV/XV.
Now *Vaticanus Barberinianus graecus* 566 (*Census*: 273, nr [1436]).

Nemesius Emesenus: (f. 71) *De natura hominis* (Frgm.).

Rom, Bibl. Barberin., 382 (I 91); s. XV.
Same as **I 91 (382)** above (p. 146).
= *Vaticanus Barberinianus graecus* 91 (*Census*: 274, nr [1439]).

Rufus: (f. 27^{v}) *De vesicae renumque affectibus.*

Rom, Bibl. Corsiniana (= Acc. d. Lincei)
Now Roma, Biblioteca Corsiniana, Accademia dei Lincei

Rom, Bibl. Corsiniana (= Acc. d. Lincei), 14 (Rossi 358); s. –.
Now *Corsin.* 43.D.32 (*Census*: 274, nr [1440]).

Diodorus: (f. 11) *De mensuris et ponderibus.*

Rom, Bibl. Vallicellana
Roma, Biblioteca Vallicelliana

Rom, Bibl. Vallicellana, – (Allatianus); s. –.
= *Allatianus* VI (*Census*: 275, nr [1444]).

Nepualius: *De sympathicis et antipathicis.*

Rom, Bibl. Vallicellana, 15 (B 70); s. XIV (XV).
Now B 70 (*Census*: 276, nr [1445]).

Alexander Trallianus: *Therapeutica. Libri XII* (L. I usque ad τὸ ἰνίον ὀδύνωνται πολλάκις· ἐὰν δὲ ...).

Rom, Bibl. Vallicellana, 78 (F 9); s. XVI.
Now F 9 (*Census*: 276, nr [1447]).

Erotianus: (f. 188–196ᵛ) *Vocum Hippocraticarum conlectio* (Expl. παρὰ τὸ δόρυ^ει παύειν· ὃ γὰρ ἡμεῖς).

Rom, Bibl. Vaticana, Ottobon.
Now Città del Vaticano, Biblioteca Apostolica Vaticana, *Ottoboniani*

Rom, Bibl. Vaticana, Ottobon. 89; s. XVI.
See also **Vatic. – (Puschm. I p. 89)** below (p. 154).

Alexander Trallianus: (f. 1) *Therapeutica. Libri XII.*

Rom, Bibl. Vaticana, Ottobon. 129; s. XVII.

Oribasius:
(f. 1) *Conspectus ad Eustathium filium. Libri II.*
(f. 38) *Ad Eunapium de parabilibus medicamentis. Libri IV.*

Rom, Bibl. Vaticana, Ottobon. 145; a. 1363.

Meletius monachus: (f. 1) *De natura hominis.*

Rom, Bibl. Vaticana, Ottobon. 192; s. XVI–XVII.

Soranus: (f. 285) *Excerpta varia* (Σωρανὸς ὁ Ζωγράγος).

Rom, Bibl. Vaticana, Ottobon. 235; s. –.
Same as **Rom, Fonds Colonna, 12** below (p. 164) (*Census*: 277, nr [1456]).

Rufus: (f. 1) *De corporis humani appellationibus.*
Oribasius: (f. 17) *Medicae collectiones ad Iulianum* (L. XXIV–XXV 58).

Rom, Bibl. Vaticana, Ottobon. 259; s. XIV–XV.

Epiphanius: (f. 122) *De mensuris et ponderibus.*

Rom, Bibl. Vaticana, Ottobon. 275; s. XVII.

Nemesius Emesenus: (f. 76) *De natura hominis* (Frgm.).

Rom, Bibl. Vaticana, Ottobon. 311; s. XV–XVI, XVI.

Stephanus Atheniensis: (f. 79) *De febrium differentiis ex ore Theophili.*
Aëtius Amidenus: (f. 95ᵛ) *Iatricorum libri XVI* (L. II).
Theodorus: (f. 117ᵛ) *Excerpta* (Θεραπεία εἰς ἐπιληπτικοὺς καταπίποντας, ἐκ τοῦ δευτέρου Θεοδώρου).

Rom, Bibl. Vaticana, Ottobon. 441; a. 1477.

Asclepiades: (f. 476) *Praecepta salubria.*

Rom, Bibl. Vaticana, Ottobon. 464; s. XVI.

Nemesius Emesenus: (f. 1) *De natura hominis.*

Rom, Bibl. Vaticana, Palat.
Now Città del Vaticano, Biblioteca Apostolica Vaticana, *Palatini*

Rom, Bibl. Vaticana, Palat. 13; a. 1167.

Splenius philosophus: (f. 347ᵛ) *De gemeratione hominis* (Sine auct. nom.).

Rom, Bibl. Vaticana, Palat. 48; s. XVI.

Dioscurides:
(f. 1) *De materia medica* (Lib. II 54 – VIII).
(f. 166ᵛ) *De venenis eorumque praecautione et medicatione.*
(f. 177) *De iis, quae virus eiaculantur, animalibus libellus, in quo et de rabioso cane.*
Andromachus: (f. 192) *Theriaca.*

Rom, Bibl. Vaticana, Palat. 77; s. XIV.

Dioscurides:
De venenis eorumque praecautione et medicatione.
De iis, quae virus eiaculantur, animalibus libellus, in quo et de rabioso cane.
(f. 1) *Excerpta.*
Neophytus Prodromenus: (f. 3) *Remediorum collectio alphabetica.*
Dioscurides: (f. 15) *De materia medica* (Libri I–IX).

Rom, Bibl. Vaticana, Palat. 199; s. XIII.

Oribasius: (f. 16^{v}) *Excerpta varia* (Περὶ μέτρων καὶ σταθμῶν ἰατρικῶν. Inc. Ὁ μέδιμνος ἔχει [M. W.]).
Neophytus Prodromenus: (f. 17) *Remediorum collectio alphabetica* (Λέξις βοτανῶν κατὰ στοιχεῖον ἀλφαβήτου. Inc. Ἄρκευστον ἢ καντζάρου ἢ κέδρος).
Alexander Aphrodisiensis: (f. 18) *Problematum physicorum et medicorum eclogae. Libri V.*
Aëtius Amidenus: (f. 101) *Iatricorum libri XVI* (Libri IX, omisso l. VII, de ocularibus morbis. *Nach Zervos L. I–XI, ohne VII*).
Oribasius: *Excerpta varia*:
(f. 149^{v} sq.) (folgende Capitel, die = Orib. I 436 ff.: περὶ κατακλίσεως, ἐκ τῶν Ἀντύλλου καὶ Γαληνοῦ ἐκ τῶν ποιουμένων βοηθημάτων, περὶ ἡσυχίας ἐκ τοῦ αὐτοῦ λόγου, περὶ ἀσιτίας ἐκ τοῦ αὐτοῦ λόγου, περὶ ὕπνου καὶ ἐγρηγόρεως Γαληνοῦ, περὶ τῆς ἐξ ὕπνου ὠφελείας Ἀντύλλου, περὶ ἐγρηγόρεως τοῦ αὐτοῦ, περὶ λαλιᾶς τοῦ αὐτοῦ. Dann περὶ τῶν μέσων ἐδεσμάτων τῶν αὐτῶν Γαληνοῦ = Orib. I 173. Dann folgen die weitern Capitel Orib. I 174. 177. 182. 178 [M. W.]).
(f. 168^{v}) Περὶ λουτρῶν σαφὲς = Orib. II 369 [M. W.].
(f. 181^{v}) Περὶ τῶν ἐν τοῖς συμπτώμασιν αἰτίων = Orib. III 208. Daran schließen sich weitere Excerpte bis fol. 183^{v} [M. W.].
Rufus: (f. 181^{v}) *De medicamentis purgantibus* (Περὶ καθάρσεως τῆς κατὰ κοιλίαν πρόγνωσις Ῥούφου Ἐφεσίου = Orib. II 94f. [M. W.]).
Theophilus: (f. 190) *De arte medica, ex Hippocrate et Galeno* (Expl. ἀποτελεῖται ἀπὸ τῆς μήτρας [M. W.]).

Rom, Bibl. Vaticana, Palat. 226; s. XV.
See also (possibly) **[Vatic.]** below (p. 154).

Hermes Trismegistus: *Kyranides*.

Rom, Bibl. Vaticana, Palat. 279; s. XIV–XV.

Paulus Aegineta: *Excerpta varia:*
(f. 212^{v}) De phlebotomia, exc. ex Galeno et Paulo Aeg. Inc. Οἱ πρῶτοι καὶ κυριώτατοι σκοποὶ τῆς φλεβοτομίας.
(f. 214^{v}) Π. φλεβοτομίας. Inc. Ὁ τῆς φλεβοτομίας τρόπος).
Magnus Emesenus: (f. 292) *De urinis* (»f. 280^{v} idem liber contractior«).
Aëtius Amidenus: (f. 312^{v}) *Excerpta varia* (De febrium diagnosi et curatione).

Rom, Bibl. Vaticana, Palat. 297; s. XV–XVI.

Palladius: *Stephani philosophi vel Palladii synopsis de febribus* (Ex Galeno de febrium substantia et differentiis praevio indice. *Vgl.* [Flor.] Laurent. 74, 11 [above p. 44]. Inc. prol. Σκοπὸν οὖν ἔχομεν).

Rom, Bibl. Vaticana, Palat. 302; s. XVI.

Rufus: (f. 40) *De corporis humani appellationibus.*

Rom, Bibl. Vaticana, Palat. 328; s. XV.

Splenius philosophus: (f. 154ᵛ) *De generatione hominis* (Π. γενέσ. ἀνθρ. Σπλ. φιλοσ.).

Rom, Bibl. Vaticana, Palat. 358; s. XV–XVI.

Aëtius Amidenus: (f. 230) *Excerpta varia* (De capillorum defluvio. Inc. Περὶ τὸ μὴ ἀπορρεῖν τρίχας).

Rom, Bibl. Vaticana, Palat. 370; s. XV.

Nemesius Emesenus: (f. 1ᵛ) *De natura hominis.*
Ioannes Zacharias Actuarius: (f. 151) *De methodo medendi libri VI* (L. IV. V).

Rom, Bibl. Vaticana, Palat. 375; s. XII.

Oribasius: (f. 230) *Medicae collectiones ad Iulianum* (L. XXIV. XXV).

Rom, Bibl. Vaticana, Palat. 385; s. XV–XVI.

Nemesius Emesenus: (f. 121) *De natura hominis.*

Rom, Bibl. Vaticana, Palat. 400; s. XV.

Herophilus: (f. 60ᵛ) *De febricantibus.*
Herophilus Sophista:
(f. 75) *De alimentis, quae singulis mensibus sumenda aut vitanda sunt* (Inc. Ταύτης τῆς ἐπιτρέψεως).
(f. 83ᵛ) *De alimentorum facultatibus.*
Meletius monachus: (f. 146ᵛ) *De natura hominis.*
Paulus Aegineta: (f. 383) *Excerpta varia* (Simplicium et compositorum pharmacorum experimenta).

Dioscurides:
(f. 383) *De facile parabilibus tam simplicibus quam compositis medicamentis libri II* (Frgm. Palat. 400 »ist zu streichen«. M. W.).
(f. 383) *Excerpta varia* (»Βιβλίον Διοσκ. · αὕτη ἡ βίβλος περιέχει τέχνην πείρας ἰατρικῆς περὶ ἁπλῶν τε καὶ συνθέτων φαρμάκων κατὰ ἀλφάβητον ὑποτεταγμένων κτλ.« M. W.).

Rom, Bibl. Vaticana, Palat. 428; s. XV–XVI, XV–XVII.

Index: (f. 1) Index in Gal., **Alex. Aphr.** et Hipp. aliquot opuscola.
Diocles: (f. 26) *Ad Antigonum regem epistula de tuenda valetitudine.*

Rom, Bibl. Vaticana, Reg. Suec.
Now Città del Vaticano, Biblioteca Apostolica Vaticana, *Reginenses*

Rom, Bibl. Vaticana, Reg. Suec. 176; s. XIV.

Paulus Aegineta: (f. 2) *Epitomae medicae libri septem.*
Palladius: (f. 302) *De cibo et potione.*

Rom, Bibl. Vaticana, Reg. Suec. 181; a. 1364.
See also (possibly) **Vatic. 1052** below (p. 160).

Ioannes Zacharias Actuarius: (f. 1) *De methodo medendi libri VI* (L. I–V).

Rom, Bibl. Vaticana, Reg. Suec. 182; s. XV.

Ioannes Esdra: (f. 4) *De urinis.*

Rom, Bibl. Vaticana, Urbin.
Now Città del Vaticano, Biblioteca Apostolica Vaticana, *Urbinates*

Rom, Bibl. Vaticana, Urbin. 64; s. X–XI, XIII.

Galenos (*Ist der Commentar des* **Palladius** *unter den Namen des* Galen): (f. 48v) *Scholia in Hippocratis de popularibus morbis librum sextum, sectiones VIII* (Σχόλιον τῆς ἕκτης ἐπιδημίας ἀπὸ φωνῆς Γαλ. VII partes. Inc. Ἄρτι ταῖς μεθόδοις τὰ ὀξέα τῶν νοσημάτων).
Palladius (sub Galeni nomine): (f. 94) *Scholia in Hippocratis de popularibus morbis librum sextum, sectiones VIII.*

Rom, Bibl. Vaticana, Urbin. 66; s. XV.

Dioscurides:
(f. 1–120) *De materia medica* (Inscr. Περὶ παντὸς εἴδους βοτανῶν καὶ ῥιζῶν καὶ τῶν θεραπειῶν αὐτῶν. alphab.).
(f. 146–155) *De venenis eorumque praecautione et medicatione* (Inscr. *wie im* Athous [Βιβλ. Μον. Λαύρας Ω 75] [above p. 11]).
(f. 155) *De iis, quae virus eiaculantur, animalibus libellus, in quo et de rabioso cane.*
(f. 165ᵛ) *Metaphrasis in Nicandri Theriaca et Alexipharmaca.*
Eutecnius:
(f. 165ᵛ) *Paraphrasis in Nicandri Theriaca.*
(f. 183) *Paraphrasis in Nicandri Alexipharmaca.*
(f. 193ᵛ) *Paraphrasis in Oppiani Halieutica* (Inc. Ταῖς ῥαφίσιν δὲ ὡς λεπταῖς διεξελθεῖν. Expl. ὥσπερ οὐδὲ τῶν παστάδων αἱ γυναῖκες).

Rom, Bibl. Vaticana, Urbin. 67; s. XIII, XIV, XIV–XV, XV.

Hermes Trismegistus: (f. 186ᵛ) *Excerpta varia* (»Ἀντίδοτος πρὸς ποδαλγικοὺς πάνυ πεπειραμένη αἰγυπτιακὴ τρισμέγιστος, φοβερὰ δόκιμος γεναμένη εἰς ὑγείαν πολλῶν ἀνθρώπων.« M. W.).
Syncellus: (f. 187) *Excerpta* (Ἀντίδοτος τοῦ Συγκέλλου. [M. W.]).

Rom, Bibl. Vaticana, Urbin. 68; s. XIV.

Erotianus: *Vocum Hippocraticarum conlectio.*
Soranus: (f. 4) *Hippocratis genus et vita secundum Soranum.*

Rom, Bibl. Vaticana, Urbin. 70; s. XV.

Rufus, Posidonius, Marcellus: (f. 107) *De melancholia ex Galeno, Rufo, Posidonio et Marcello Sicamii Aetii libellus.*
Aëtius Amidenus: (f. 107) *Excerpta varia* (Π. μελαγχολίας ἐκ τῶν Γαλ. καὶ Ῥουφ. καὶ Ποσειδ.).

Rom, Bibl. Vaticana, Urbin. 158; s. XIII.

Paulus Aegineta: (f. 269) *Excerpta varia* (Σύντομοι καὶ εὐσύνοπτοι ἰατρεῖαι διαφόρων νοσημάτων).

Rom, Bibl. Vaticana, Vatic.
Now Città del Vaticano, Biblioteca Apostolica Vaticana, *Vaticani graeci*

Rom, Bibl. Vaticana, Vatic. *bei Migne.*
= *Vaticanus graecus* 434 (*Census*: 284, nr [1510]).

S. Basilius: *Ad Eusthatum medicum de obiectionum haereticorum solutione.*

[Rom, Bibl. Vaticana, Vatic.].
Possibly *Vaticanus Palatinus graecus* 226 above (p. 150) (*Census*: 284, nr [1511]).

Harpocration: *De facultatibus naturalibus animalium et herbarum et lapidum.*

Rom, Bibl. Vaticana, Vatic. – (Puschm. I p. 89).
= *Vaticanus Ottobonianus* 89 above (p. 148) (*Census*: 285, nr [1512]).

Alexander Trallianus: *Epistula de lumbricis.*

Rom, Bibl. Vaticana, Vatic. 12; s. XIV.

Splenius philosophus: (f. 206^{v}) *De generatione hominis* (Inscr. Π. γεν. ἀνθρ. ὅθεν τά τε τρίτα καὶ ἔννατα καὶ τὰ τεσσαρακοστά).
Rufus:
(f. 236^{v}) *De dissectione partium corporis humani* (Frgm. *Vgl.* Daremberg p. 236).
(f. 236^{v}) *Excerpta varia* (*Vgl.* Daremb. p. 236).
(f. 236^{v}) *Nomenclatura rerum ad hominem pertinentium. Libri III* (*Vgl.* Daremb. p. 236).

Rom, Bibl. Vaticana, Vatic. 178; s. XIV.

Archigenes: (f. 142^{v}) *Excerpta* (Περὶ συναπισμοῦ. Inc. Τὸ ἀπὸ νάπυος. Expl. καταχύσει παρηγορητέον).

Rom, Bibl. Vaticana, Vatic. 277; s. XIV.

Erotianus: (f. 2) *Vocum Hippocraticarum conlectio.*
Soranus: (f. 24) *Hippocratis genus et vita secundum Soranum.*

Rom, Bibl. Vaticana, Vatic. 278; a. 1512.

Soranus: (f. 25^{v}) *Hippocratis genus et vita secundum Soranum.*

Rom, Bibl. Vaticana, Vatic. 279; s. –, XII.
Verbleib unbekannt.
See *Census*: 290–291, nr [1524].

Magnus Emesenus: (f. 176ᵛ) *De febribus.*
Paulus Aegineta: (f. 214) *Excerpta varia* (Π. φλεβοτομίας. »Hic codex deest«; *Verwechslung mit dem* Palat. 279? [above p. 150]).
Magnus Emesenus:
(f. 280) *Prognosticon.*
(f. 280) *De urinis.*

Rom, Bibl. Vaticana, Vatic. 280; s. XV.

Romanus: (f. 162ᵛ) *De morbis acutis et chronicis* (Ῥωμανοῦ καὶ κουβουκλησίου τῆς τοῦ Θεοῦ ἐκκλησίας ἁγίας καὶ πτορομηνιτου [sic] τοῦ βασιλικοῦ ξενῶνος τοῦ μυρελαίου καὶ τῆς περιδόξου. Inc. Οὐ παραιτητέον. Expl. αἷς ὑγιεινόν ἐστιν).
Magnus Emesenus: (f. 176ᵛ) *De urinis* (*Vgl.* Ideler I p. 283).
Theophilus: (f. 197ᵛ) *De alvi excrementis* (Fine mutil.; expl. 408, 1 Idel.).
Ioannes Philoponus Alexandrinus: (f. 204) *De pulsibus.*
Meletius monachus: (f. 212) *De natura hominis.*

Rom, Bibl. Vaticana, Vatic. 282; s. XV.
s. XVI.

Aëtius Amidenus: (f. 146) *Iatricorum libri XVI* (L. VI–XVI).
Ioannes Staphidaces: (f. 433) *De nonnullorum medicamentorum compositione* (»Σύνθεσις ἀκριβὴς διαφόρων πράξεων ἐκβληθεῖσα καὶ συντεθεῖσα ὡς ἀναγκαῖον [in mg. ἰωάννου τοῦ σταφιδάκη]. Inc. Κουφότερον καθαρτικόν · ἐπιθύμου ςΓ δ' · μυροβάλατα ςΓ η'. Expl. f. 444ᵛ ἔχον τὴν σαμίαν αἰγυπτίαν ῥόδα.« M. W.).

Rom, Bibl. Vaticana, Vatic. 283; s. XIV.

Palladius: (f. 16ᵛ) *Stephani philosophi vel Palladii synopsis de febribus.*

Rom, Bibl. Vaticana, Vatic. 284; s. XI–XII (?), XII.
s. XI.

Dioscurides:
Excerpta varia (»Was über ihn hier gesagt ist, kann jetzt wegfallen.« M. W.).
(f. 1) *De materia medica* (»Enthält eine illustrierte Compilation aus Gal. περὶ δυνάμεως φαρμάκων und D. περὶ ὕλης ἰατρικῆς, nach der galenischen Schrift geordnet; vorn unvollständig, umfaßt sie Gal. l. VI–XI. Inc. ρ̅μ̅

περὶ δράβεως: – ⟨δράβη ἡ⟩ πόα. Expl. f. 251ʳ Γαληνοῦ τῶν ἁπλῶν βιβλίον ια' ἐπληρώθη ἔχον ἀπὸ τοῦ Διοσκουρίδου ὅσα Γαληνῷ παραλέλειπται.« M. W.).

(f. 1–251, 251ᵛ) *Excerpta* (Γαλ. τῶν ἁπλῶν βιβλίον ϛ'–ια' ἔχον ἀπὸ τοῦ Δ. ὅσα Γαληνῷ παραλέλειπται *und* f. 251ᵛ Κεφάλαια τῶν ἐν τῷ ϛ' βιβλίῳ Δ.).

(f. 251ᵛ) *De venenis eorumque praecautione et medicatione.*

(f. 252) *De materia medica* (Liber VI).

Philumenus: (f. 264ᵛ) *De venenatis animalibus* (Περὶ ἰοβόλων ζῴων καὶ τῶν ἐν αὐτοῖς βοηθημάτων).

Dioscurides: (f. 265) *De iis, quae virus eiaculantur, animalibus libellus, in quo et de rabioso cane* (Frgm. Inc. Γνήσιον καὶ ὠφέλιμον ἐφάνη μοι. Expl. ἑξῆς τὰ λοιπά, mutil. in fine).

Africanus: (f. 288ᵛ) *Ex Africani Cestis cestum XIII cap. 22: De purgantibus simplicibus* (Ἐκ τῶν Ἀ. κεστῶν περὶ τοῦ κιναμώμου. M. W.).

Rom, Bibl. Vaticana, Vatic. 285; s. XV.

Stephanus Atheniensis: (f. 196) *De febrium differentiis ex ore Theophili.*

Herophilus Sophista: (f. 301) *De alimentis, quae singulis mensibus sumenda aut vitanda sunt.*

Rom, Bibl. Vaticana, Vatic. 286; s. XV.

Aretaeus:

(f. 1) *De causis et signis acutorum morborum libri II* (ab initio mutil.).

(f. 32ᵛ) *De causis et signis diuturnorum morborum libri II.*

(f. 92) *De curatione acutorum morborum libri II.*

(f. 145) *De curatione diuturnorum morborum libri II* (Expl. in med. c. 5).

Rom, Bibl. Vaticana, Vatic. 287; s. XV.

Oribasius: (f. 1) *Conspectus ad Eustathium filium. Libri II.*

Rom, Bibl. Vaticana, Vatic. 288; s. XV.

Oribasius: (f. 1) *Medicae collectiones ad Iulianum* (L. I–XV).

Rom, Bibl. Vaticana, Vatic. 289; s. XIV–XV, XV.

Dioscurides:

(f. 5) *De materia medica* (Libri VII).

(f. 98) *De venenis eorumque praecautione et medicatione.*

(f. 102) *De iis, quae virus eiaculantur, animalibus libellus, in quo et de rabioso cane.*

Rom, Bibl. Vaticana, Vatic. 290; s. XVI.

Dioscurides: (f. 1) *De facile parabilibus tam simplicibus quam compositis medicamentis libri II* (»stammt aus [Florent.] Laurent. 74, 20 [above p. 45].« M. W.).

Rom, Bibl. Vaticana, Vatic. 291; s. XV–XVI.

Rufus:
(f. 1) *De vesicae renumque affectibus* (*Vgl.* Mai, Classici auct. IV. p. 198).
(f. 20) *Nomenclatura rerum ad hominem pertinentium. Libri III* (*Vgl.* Dbg.-R. praef. p. XXV).

Rom, Bibl. Vaticana, Vatic. 293; s. XVI.

Ioannes Episcopus Prisdianensis: (f. 22) *Collectanea de urinis* (Συντάξεις θεοφόρου ἀνδρὸς καὶ ἐπισκόπου Ἰωάννου περὶ οὔρων καὶ ἄλλων πολλῶν).

Rom, Bibl. Vaticana, Vatic. 294; s. –.

Paulus Aegineta: (f. 296) *Excerpta varia* (Π. ἀντιβαλλομένων).

Rom, Bibl. Vaticana, Vatic. 295; s. XV.

Antyllus: *Excerpta* (Περὶ πεσσῶν).
Paulus Aegineta: (f. 1) *Epitomae medicae libri septem.*

Rom, Bibl. Vaticana, Vatic. 296; s. XV.

Paulus Aegineta: (f. 1) *Epitomae medicae libri septem.*

Rom, Bibl. Vaticana, Vatic. 297; s. XIV.

Aëtius Amidenus: (f. 1) *Iatricorum libri XVI* (»enthalten Buch I–XVI.« M. W.).

Rom, Bibl. Vaticana, Vatic. 298; a. 1387.

Aëtius Amidenus: (f. 5) *Iatricorum libri XVI* (»enthalten Buch I–XVI.« M. W.).
Africanus: (f. 591) *De ponderibus et mensuris.*

Rom, Bibl. Vaticana, Vatic. 299; s. XV.

Ioannes Zacharias Actuarius:
(f. 17) *Tractatus de urinis, qui ex Avicenna translatus dicitur in graecam linguam a Christodulo, in ordinem redactus ab Actuario Zacharia.*

(f. 20ᵛ) *De urinis libri VII.*

Mercurius monachus: (f. 101) *De pulsibus* (»Inc. Τὸ σῶμα τοῦ ἀνθρώπου συνέστηκεν ἐκ δ' στοιχείων. Expl. f. 101ᵛ κατὰ λέξιν τοιόνδε.« M. W.).

Manuel Comnenus: (f. 131) *De compositione medicamentorum* (»Τῶν σκευασιῶν ἡ βίβλος αὕτη πέλει καὶ δυναμερὸν σὺν θεῷ λεγομένη. Ἀρχὴ καὶ πρώτη σκευασία τῆς θηριακῆς. Es folgt Index von ος' Kapiteln und Index der σκευασίαι τῶν ἐμπλάστρων mit οθ' Kapiteln. Text beginnt f. 132 mit Überschrift: π' σκευασία τοῦ ζουλαπίου κυρίου Μανουὴλ Κομνηνοῦ · σκευασία τῆς θηριακῆς).

Lucas: (f. 148) *Compositio salsi intinctus* (»Ἁλάτιον σκευασθὲν ὑπὸ τοῦ ἁγίου ἀποστόλου Λουκᾶ ἔχον ἐνεργείας τῶν ὑποτεταγμένων κεφαλαίων. Expl. ἐν αὐτῷ τὰς τροφὰς πάσας.« M. W.).

Paulus Aegineta:

(f. 153ᵛ) *Epitomae medicae libri septem* (L. VII 26).

(f. 153ᵛ) *De succedaneis* (M. W.).

Aëtius Amidenus: (f. 156) *Excerpta varia* (Κόμητος τοῦ ὀψικίου ἐκ τῶν ἁπλῶν Γαλ. Inc. Ἀδιάφοροι τῶν κατὰ μέρος. Expl. καὶ μάλιστα νήπια; »Ist B. I.« M. W.).

Democritus: (f. 309–314ᵛ. 329. 366ᵛ. 391) *Excerpta varia* (Varia capita Pseudo-Democritea; *vgl.* E. Rohde, Kl. Schr. I p. 383 adn.).

Eustathius: (f. 393ᵛ) *Excerpta* (»Commemoratur ἐγὼ Εὐστάθιος ὁ εὐτελὴς ἰατρός«).

Dioscurides: (f. 449ᵛ) *De mensuris et ponderibus* (Frgm. Inc. Τὸ κεράτιον τῷ αὐτῷ. Expl. ὁ κύαθος ⌈ο α' <ε ⌈ᵖ '' α').

Aelius Promotus: (f. 451) *Dynameron* (Inc. Τὰ λείποντα ἀπὸ τοῦ νη' κεφαλαίου ἐκ τοῦ βιβλίου τοῦ Προμώτου · ἄλλο βαπτικόν · κικίδα < δ'. »Diese Excerpte stammen aus cap. ρε' ff. des Δυναμερόν.« M. W.).

Heliodorus: (f. 451) *De mensuris et ponderibus.*

Aelius Promotus:

(f. 473–493ᵛ) *De animalibus virus eiculantibus* (*Abschrift im Berol. 39 [275]* [above p. 15]).

(f. 494–495ᵛ) *Physica et antipathetica.*

Nepualius: (f. 495 b) *De sympathicis et antipathicis.*

Democritus: (f. 498) *De sympathicis et antipathicis.*

Rom, Bibl. Vaticana, Vatic. 300; s. XII–XIII.

Gregorius Theologus: (f. 293) *De compositione et distinctione corporis humani* (Inc. Δεύτερον ἐννοεῖ κόσμον. Expl. στοιχεῖα τοῦ ἀνθρώπου).

Rom, Bibl. Vaticana, Vatic. 423; s. X.

Nemesius Emesenus: (f. 227ᵛ) *De natura hominis* (Inc. Τὸν ἄνθρωπον ἴσμεν. Expl. τῆς αὐτοῦ βασιλείας. Frgm.?).

Rom, Bibl. Vaticana, Vatic. 429; s. XV–XVI.

Ioannes Zacharias Actuarius: (f. 315) *De spiritu animali libri II* (*Nur* liber II?).
Taronitus (?): (f. 341ᵛ) *Excerpta* (Κατάστοιχον εἰς δυσουρίαν. Inc. Ἀλθαίας σπέρματα. Expl. μέλιτος τὸ ἀρκοῦν).

Rom, Bibl. Vaticana, Vatic. 489; s. XV–XVI.

Nemesius Emesenus: (f. 3) *De natura hominis*.

Rom, Bibl. Vaticana, Vatic. 517 (*Vgl.* Costomiris, Rev. des ét. gr. X [1897] p. 435).

Ioannes Zacharias Actuarius: *Opera*.

Rom, Bibl. Vaticana, Vatic. 578; s. XV.

Orpheus: *De lapidibus*.

Rom, Bibl. Vaticana, Vatic. 671; s. XIII–XIV.

Ioannes Pothus Pediasimus: (f. 237) Τοῦ ὑπάτου τῶν φιλοσόφων κυρίου ἰωάννου πόθου τοῦ πεδιασίμου. Inc. Ἐζήτηται δι' ἣν αἰτίαν ἐννιάμηνος μὲν τόκος. Expl. ἀλλ' ἀρκοῦσι ταῦτα.

Rom, Bibl. Vaticana, Vatic. 695; s. XIV–XV.

Epiphanius: *Physiologus* (Inc. Ὁ φυσιολόγος ἔλεξε περὶ τοῦ ἐλέφαντος).

Rom, Bibl. Vaticana, Vatic. 854; s. XI.

Splenius philosophus: (f. 265ᵛ) *De generatione hominis* (Sine auct. nomine).

Rom, Bibl. Vaticana, Vatic. 855; s. XVI.

Splenius philosophus: (f. 312ᵛ) *De generatione hominis* (Sine auctor. nomine. Expl. mutil. τῆς ἐπιρροῆς καὶ θηλύ⟨νεται⟩).

Rom, Bibl. Vaticana, Vatic. 876; s. XV.

Oribasius: (f. 3) *Excerpta varia* (*Wie im* [Flor.] Laurent. [plut. 74, 7] [above p. 42]. *Vgl.* Dbg.-Buss. I p. XXXV).

Rom, Bibl. Vaticana, Vatic. 952; s. XIV.

Hermes Trismegistus: (f. 184ᵛ) *Canon*.

Rom, Bibl. Vaticana, Vatic. 1052 (*Vgl.* Costomiris, Rev. des ét. gr. X [1897] p. 435).
Possibly same as *Vaticanus Reginensis graecus* 181 above (p. 152) (*Census*: 297, nr [1558]).

Ioannes Zacharias Actuarius: *Opera.*

Rom, Bibl. Vaticana, Vatic. 1062; s. XVI.

Theophilus: (f. 1) *Commentarius in Hippocratis aphorismos.*

Rom, Bibl. Vaticana, Vatic. 1066; s. XVI.
s. XV.

Hermes Trismegistus: (f. 18ᵛ) *Methodus ad omne inceptum idonea.*

Rom, Bibl. Vaticana, Vatic. 1133 (1134 Kl.); s. –, XVII.
= *Vaticanus graecus* 1133 (*Census*: 298, nr [1565]).

Erotianus: *Vocum Hippocraticarum conlectio* (Apogr. codicis [*Vat. gr.*] 277 [above p. 154]).

Rom, Bibl. Vaticana, Vatic. 1174; s. XIV–XV.

Democritus: *Excerpta varia*:
(f. 1) Ἐκ τῶν Δημοκρίτου φυσικῶν καὶ μυστικῶν; Inc. Ἡ φύσις τῇ φύσει τέρπεται. [M. W.].
(f. 32ᵛ) Ὁ δὲ Δημόκριτος ἐκ τούτων λαβὼν συνεγράψατο βιβλία δ' τῷ τῆς ἀφορμῆς ὀνόματι κτλ. [M. W.].
(f. 33) Περὶ πορφύρας φυσικῆς.
(f. 33ᵛ) Ἐκ τῶν Δ. περὶ πορφύρας φυσικῆς. Inc. Βαλὼν εἰς λίτραν α' ποφρύρας. [M. W.].
Zosimus Panopolita: (f. 42) *De instrumentis et fornacibus.*
Stephanus Alexandrinus: (f. 54) *De magna sacraque scientia solis itineris ad regem Heraclium.*
Heliodorus: (f. 68ᵛ) *Ad Theodosium regem.*
Stephanus Alexandrinus: (f. 70ᵛ) *Epistula ad Theodorum.*
Synesius: (f. 79) *Ad Dioscorum, scholia in librum Democriti.*
Cleopatra: (f. 134ᵛ) *De mensuris et ponderibus.*

Rom, Bibl. Vaticana, Vatic. 1191 & 1194 (*Vgl.* Costomiris, Rev. des ét. gr. X [1897] p. 435).

Ioannes Zacharias Actuarius: *Opera.*

Rom, Bibl. Vaticana, Vatic. 1277; s. XV–XVI.

Splenius philosophus: (f. 55) *De generatione hominis* (Sine auct. nomine).

Rom, Bibl. Vaticana, Vatic. 1343; s. XV.

Asclepiades: (f. 2) *Praecepta salubria* (Expl. καύματος χρόνῳ).

Rom, Bibl. Vaticana, Vatic. 1347; s. XV–XVI.

Soranus: (f. 1) *De ponderibus et mensuris.*

Rom, Bibl. Vaticana, Vatic. 1427; s. XVI.

Oribasius:
(f. 1) *Conspectus ad Eustathium filium. Libri II* (Frgm.).
(f. 70) *Ad Eunapium de parabilibus medicamentis. Libri IV* (Expl. in cap. Ἐφημέρων πυρετῶν ἰάσεις).

Rom, Bibl. Vaticana, Vatic. 1444; s. XVI.
See *Census*: 300, nr [1576].

Hermes Trismegistus: (f. 217) *Iatromathematica ad Ammonium Aegyptium.*
Pancharius: (f. 235ᵛ) *Compendium de decubitu infirmorum.*
Theophilus: (f. 243ᵛ) *De principiis mundi collectanea.*

Rom, Bibl. Vaticana, Vatic. 1470; s. XIII.

Craton: (f. 158) *Prognostica de infirmorum vita et morte.*

Rom, Bibl. Vaticana, Vatic. 1614; s. XVI.

Alexander Aphrodisiensis: (f. 1) *Quarundam difficultatum solutiones* (Σχολίων ἀποριῶν καὶ λύσεων κεφάλαια τοῦ Α' λόγου).
Cassius iatrosophistes: (f. 153) *Quaestiones medicae et problemata physica.*

Rom, Bibl. Vaticana, Vatic. 1692 B; s. XV.
= *Vaticanus graecus* 1702 (*Census*: 301, nr [1581]).

Hermes Trismegistus: (f. 1) *Iatromathematica ad Ammonium Aegyptium.*
Alexander Aphrodisiensis: (f. 34) *Excerpta varia* (Περὶ τῆς ἡρακλείας λίθου καὶ διὰ τί ἕλκει τὸν σίδηρον. Inc. Ἐμπεδοκλῆς ταῖς ἀποῤῥοίαις. Expl. τῶν ἀψύχων ἔχει. Ex libro II quaest. naturalium?).

Rom, Bibl. Vaticana, Vatic. 1695; s. XV.

Meletius monachus: (f. 1) *De natura hominis.*

Rom, Bibl. Vaticana, Vatic. 1835; s. –.

Oribasius: *Medicae collectiones ad Iulianum* (L. XLIV–LI).

Rom, Bibl. Vaticana, Vatic. 1879; s. XV.

Soranus: (f. 159) *Hippocratis genus et vita secundum Soranum.*

Rom, Bibl. Vaticana, Vatic. 1885; s. XIV.

Oribasius: (f. 1) *Medicae collectiones ad Iulianum* (Frgm. Inc. Τῶν τοιούτων ... αὐτῷ μέν. *Vgl.* A. Mai, Auctor. class. IV p. 276–278).
Heliodorus: (f. 2) *Excerpta varia* (Περὶ τῶν ἐν κατακαλύψει ἀποστημάτων. Ex Orib. III 578).
Rufus: (f. 154^{v}) *Excerpta varia* (Ἐκ τῶν Ῥούφου τοῦ Ἱππ. βάθρον ἀπὸ τῶν προοιμίων τοῦ μονοβίβλου τοῦ ἐπὶ γῆρας ἄνθρωπος, τινὲς δὲ αὐτὸ περὶ ἐξαρθημάτων ἐπιγράφουσιν. »*Stammt aus* Orib. IV 432 *mit* Scholion.« Wellmann. *Vgl.* den [Flor.] Laurent. 74, 7 [above p. 42]).

Rom, Bibl. Vaticana, Vatic. 1902; s. –.

Democritus: (f. 268) *De sympathicis et antipathicis.*

Rom, Bibl. Vaticana, Vatic. 1904; a. 1306.

Aëtius Amidenus: (f. 130) *Iatricorum libri XVI* (L. I; »enthält nur B. I und einen Teil des Index.« M. W.).
Diocles: (f. 226) *Ad Antigonum regem epistula de tuenda valetitudine.*
Dioscurides: (f. 227^{v}) *De mensuris et ponderibus.*

Rom, Bibl. Vaticana, Vatic. 1911; s. XIII.
s. XIV.

Aëtius Amidenus: (f. 1) *Iatricorum libri XVI* (L. I. II; »B. I und B. II unvollständig, schließt mit cap. ρπγ'.« M. W.).

Rom, Bibl. Vaticana, Vatic. 1949; s. –.

Africanus: (f. 198^{v}) *De ponderibus et mensuris.*

Rom, Bibl. Vaticana, Vatic. 2154; s. XVI.

Damascius: (f. 3) *Expositio in Prognostica Hippocratis. Sectiones II.*

Rom, Bibl. Vaticana, Vatic. 2182; s. XV.

Dioscurides: (f. 58) *De materia medica* (Liber III–IV, a cap. σοα' ad φοα').
Ioannes Zacharias Actuarius:
(f. 81, 89) *De urinis libri VII* (Frgm. f. 81: L. V prooem. 7–V 10, 13 = Idel. II 112–129; f. 89: L. VI pr. 6–VI 12, 10 = Idel. II 145–162).
(f. 97, 139v) *De methodo medendi Libri VI* (Inc. mutil. χείων ἡ ὑπόθεσις = Idel. I 355, 36).

Rom, Bibl. Vaticana, Vatic. 2202; s. XIV–XV.

Aëtius Amidenus: (f. 3–318) *Iatricorum libri XVI* (L. I–IV; »L. I–IV und Inhaltsverzeichnis von B. V z. T.« M. W.).

Rom, Bibl. Vaticana, Vatic. 2250; s. XIV.

Lucas: (f. 343v) *Compositio salsi intinctus.*

Rom, Bibl. Vaticana, Vatic. 2254; s. X–XI.

Theophilus: (f. 25) *Commentarius in Hippocratis aphorismos* (Sine auctor. nomine. Expl. καὶ οἷον ὑποχόνδρια μετέωρα = Dtz. II 500, 2).

Rom, Bibl. Vaticana, Vatic. 2256; s. XIV.
See *Census*: 305, nr [1601].

Rufus: (f. 26) *Excerpta varia* (Ἱερὰ υγ τῶν μελαγχολικῶν).

Rom, Bibl. Vaticana, Vatic. 2259; s. –.

Stephanus Alexandrinus:
(f. 16) *De mundo. Libri IX.*
(f. 25) *Epistula ad Theodorum.*
Cleopatra: (f. 132) *De mensuris et ponderibus.*

Rom, Bibl. Vaticana, Vatic. 2304 [olim 2217]; s. XV, XV–XVI.
Now *Vaticanus graecus* 2304 (*Census*: 306, nr [1603]).

Theophilus: (f. 1v) *De pulsibus.*
Democritus: (f. 6) *Prognosticon* (Προγν. περὶ οἰδημάτων. Inc. Οἴδημα ἄπονον περὶ τοῦ προσώπου καὶ τῆς ἀριστερᾶς χειρός. Expl. τῷ αὐτῷ χρόνῳ τελευτά. Frgm.).

Rufus: (f. 6ᵛ) *De corporis humani appellationibus* (Frgm. Inc. *wie im* [Lond. Brit. Mus.] Burneian. 94. f. 197ᵛ [above p. 64]. Expl. τῆς χειρὸς ὀνομάζονται).

Aëtius Amidenus:

(f. 8. 17–19) *Excerpta varia* (Πρόλογος περί τε δυνάμεων φυσικῶν ἐπὶ σωμάτων = Lib. I init. magni operis. f. 19: Inc. Τὸ δὲ ἀβρότονον θερμόν ἐστι. Expl. ἐν αὐτῷ τῷ ἐγκεφάλῳ ἐνισταμένης. Προεργά = pars prior libri I).

(f. 9–16ᵛ) *Excerpta varia* (f. 9: Inc. Καὶ διὰ ῥινῶν μετὰ γάλακτος. Expl. ἧπαρ ἐκκαθαίρει μὲν καὶ ῥύπτει = pars συντάγματος κατὰ στοιχεῖον π. βοτανῶν, i. e. libri I).

Rom, Bibl. Vaticana, Vatic. 3062; XVI.
= *Parisinus graecus* 3062 (*Census*: 306, nr [1604]).

Aëtius Amidenus: *Iatricorum libri XVI* (*12 Blätter*).

Rom, Bibl. Vaticana, Vatic. 3073; s. XVI.
= *Parisinus graecus* 3073 (*Census*: 306, nr [1605]).

Aëtius Amidenus: *Iatricorum libri XVI.*

Rom, Bibl. Vaticana, Vatic. 7152; –.
= *Vaticanus latinus* 7152 (*Census*: 306–307, nr [1607]).

Mercurius monachus: *De pulsibus* (*Vgl.* Daremberg *a. a. O.* [= Not. et Extr. I p. 143 sq.]).

Rom, Fonds Colonna

Rom, Fonds Colonna, 12; s. –.
= *Vaticanus Ottobonianus graecus* 235 above (p. 148) (*Census*: 269–270, nr [1417]).

Rufus: *De corporis humani appellationibus.*

Salamanca, Bibl. Univ.
Now Salamanca, Universidad de Salamanca,
Biblioteca General Histórica

Salamanca, Bibl. Univ., 1. 1. 11; a. 1524.
Now M 567 (*Census*: 309, nr [1610]).
See also (possibly) **Bibl. Univ., (Epistt. septem)** below.

Oribasius: (f. 1) *Conspectus ad Eustathium filium. Libri II.*

Salamanca, Bibl. Univ., 1. 1. 14; s. XIV.
Now M 7 (*Census*: 309, nr [1611]).

Paulus Aegineta: (f. 1) *Epitomae medicae libri septem.*

Salamanca, Bibl. Univ., (Epistt. septem).
Same as (possibly) **1. 1. 14** above (*Census*: 309, nr [1612]).
= ? M 567.

Oribasius: *Opera varia.*

Saloniki

Saloniki, Bibl. gymnas., 17; s. XIV.
Now Αθήνα, Εθνική Βιβλιοθήκη της Ελλάδος EBE 2086 (*Census*: 310, nr [1613]).

Gregorius Nyssenus: (f. 204) *De hominis opificio.*

Sáros-Patak

Sáros-Patak, Bibl. d. reform. Colleg.
= Sárospatakai Református Kollégium Todományos Gyüjteményei, Nagykönyvtár, Kt 405 (*Census*: 311, nr [1614]).

Hermes Trismegistus: *Opera* (Ἑρμους τρισμεγ. ἅπαντα. Mercurii ter maximi omnia quae exstant conquisita a. 1591).

Toledo

Toledo, Bibl. del cab. de la igl. catedr., 101, 15; s. XV.
Now Toledo Biblioteca Capitular, Catedral de Toledo, Fondo Zelada, BCT 101–15 (*Census*: 315, nr [1617]).

Harpocration: (p. 280) *De facultatibus naturalibus animalium et herbarum et lapidum* (Frgm. (Περὶ ἀσπάλαγγος. Περὶ σαλαμάνδρας).
Aëtius Amidenus: (p. 296) *Iatricorum libri XVI* (Frgm. ex l. XIII 86).

Tübingen

Tübingen, Univ.-Bibl., 2; s. XIII.
Now Mb 2 (*Census*: 316, nr [1618]).

Splenius philosophus: (f. 291) *De generatione hominis* (Σπληνίου φιλοσόφου περὶ γεννήσεως ἀνθρώπου καὶ ὅθεν τρίτα καὶ ἔννατα καὶ τεσσαρακοστὰ τοῖς τεθνεῶσιν ἐπιτελοῦσιν, παρελθόντος τοῦ ἀνθρώπου).

Turin, Bibl. Nazionale (Universitaria)
Now Torino, Biblioteca Nazionale Universitaria

Turin, Bibl. Nazionale (Universitaria), Taurinens. 6 b IV 6; s. XVI.
Now B. I. 6 (*Census*: 318, nr [1623]).

Meletius monachus: (f. 110) *De natura hominis.*

Turin, Bibl. Nazionale (Universitaria), Taurin. 156 b II 10; s. XVI.
Now C. VI. 10 (*Census*: 319, nr [1627]).

Meletius monachus: (f. 1) *De natura hominis.*
Ioannes Zacharias Actuarius: (f. 154) *Tractatus de urinis, qui ex Avicenna translatus dicitur in graecam linguam a Christodulo, in ordinem redactus ab Actuario Zacharia.*

Turin, Bibl. Nazionale (Universitaria), Taurin. 287 c I 42; s. XV.
Durch Feuer stark beschädigt.
Now C. VI. 3 (*Census*: 319, nr [1630]).

Diocles: (f. 201) *Hippocratis vel, ut alii volunt, Dioclis epistula ad Ptolemaeum Aegypti regem.*

Turin, Bibl. Nazionale (Universitaria), Taurin. C VI 21 (b VI 18); s. XVI.
= C. VI. 21 (*Census*: 320, nr [1634]).

Hermes Trismegistus: (f. 66) *Iatromathematica ad Ammonium Aegyptium* (Ἐκ τῶν ἰατρομαθηματικῶν Ἑρμοῦ καὶ Πετοσίρεως καὶ τῶν συναγωγῶν Πρωταγόρου).
Protagoras: (f. 66) *Protagorae [Pythagorae] excerpta ex iatromathematicis Mercurii et Petosiridis etc. astrologica.*

Upsala, Upsal. bibl. acad. Now Uppsala Universitet

Upsala, Upsal. bibl. acad., 8 (e don. Jo. Gabr. Sparfwenf. 49); s. –, XV.
Now Gr 8 (*Census*: 320, nr [1635]).

Paulus Aegineta: (f. 104) *Epitomae medicae libri septem* (Frgm. L. I 73 sq.).
Diocles: (f. 119) *Ad Antigonum regem epistula de tuenda valetitudine.*

Upsala, Upsal. bibl. acad., 30; s. XIII–XIV.
Now Gr 30 (*Census*: 321, nr [1637]).

Meletius monachus: *De natura hominis.*

Upsala, Upsal. bibl. acad., 34; s. XV–XVI.
Now Gr 34 (*Census*: 321, nr [1638]).

Theophilus: (f. 2) *Commentarius in Hippocratis aphorismos* (Expl. νομίζειν ἀνίατα).

Venedig, Bibl. Josephi de Aromatariis

Venedig, Bibl. Josephi de Aromatariis; s. –.
Verbleib unbekannt.
Same as **Berlin, Königl. Bibl., Phillipps. 1531 (Meerm. 223)** above (p. 17) (*Census*: 323–324, nr [1644]).
= Berlin, Staatsbibliothek zu Berlin – Preussischer Kulturbesitz SBB-PKB Ms. Phill. 1531.

Aretaeus:
De causis et signis acutorum morborum.
De causis et signis diuturnorum.

De curatione acutorum morborum.
De curatione diuturnorum morborum.

Venedig, Bibl. Josephi de Aromatariis.
Verbleib unbekannt.
Same as **Berlin, Königl. Bibl., Phillipps. 1531 (Meerm. 223)** above (p. 17) (*Census*: 325, nr [1647]).
= Berlin, Staatsbibliothek zu Berlin – Preussischer Kulturbesitz SBB-PKB Ms. Phill. 1531.

Theophilus: *De pulsibus.*

Venedig, Bibl. Nazionale Marciana, Marcian.
Now Venezia, Biblioteca Nazionale Marciana, *Marciani graeci*

Venedig, Bibl. Nazionale Marciana, graecus, 92; s. XIII.
= *Appendix graeca* XI.21 (coll. 453) (*Census*: 328–329, nr [1658]).

Paulus Aegineta: (f. 39) *De succedaneis, ex Galeno.*
Dioscurides:
(f. 92) *De venenis eorumque praecautione et medicatione* (Inscr. *wie im* Athous [Βιβλ. Μον. Λαύρας, Ω 75] [above p. 11]).
(f. 92^v) *De materia medica* (alphab.).
Crateuas: (f. 92^v) *De herbis* (Frgm. »Fragmenta continet e Vindob. med. 1 desumpta.« Wellmann).

Venedig, Bibl. Nazionale Marciana, graecus, 173; s. XIII–XIV (?).
Now *graecus* 173 (coll. 476) (*Census*: 329, nr [1659]).

Splenius philosophus: *De generatione hominis* (Sine auct. nomine. Inscr. Π. γεν. ἀνθρ. καὶ ὅθεν τρίτα καὶ θ̄ καὶ μ̄).

Venedig, Bibl. Nazionale Marciana, graecus, 257; s. XII.
Now *graecus* 257 (coll. 622) (*Census*: 329, nr [1660]).

Alexander Aphrodisiensis:
De mixtione.
Problematum physicorum et medicorum eclogae. Libri V (L. III et IV).
Cassius iatrosophistes: *Quaestiones medicae et problemata physica.*

Venedig, Bibl. Nazionale Marciana, graecus, 266; s. XV.
Now *graecus* 266 (coll. 517) (*Census*: 329, nr [1661]).

Nemesius Emesenus: (f. 99v) *De natura hominis.*

Venedig, Bibl. Nazionale Marciana, graecus, 269; s. XI.
Now *graecus* 269 (coll. 533) (*Census*: 329, nr [1662]).

Soranus: *Hippocratis genus et vita secundum Soranum.*

Venedig, Bibl. Nazionale Marciana, graecus, 270; s. XV.
Now *graecus* 270 (coll. 624) (*Census*: 329, nr [1663]).

Aretaeus:
De causis et signis acutorum morborum libri II (inc. a l. I c. 6).
De curatione acutorum morborum libri II.
De causis et signis diuturnorum morborum libri II.
De curatione diuturnorum morborum libri II.

Venedig, Bibl. Nazionale Marciana, graecus, 271; s. XV in., XV.
See also **271 (jetzt 727)** below.
Now *graecus* 271 (coll. 727) (*Census*: 329, nr [1664]).

Crateuas: *De herbis* (Frgm. Codex Dioscuridis interpolati).
Dioscurides:
De materia medica.
(f. 137) *De venenis eorumque praecautione et medicatione.*
(f. 143) *De iis, quae virus eiaculantur, animalibus libellus, in quo et de rabioso cane.*

Venedig, Bibl. Nazionale Marciana, graecus, 271 (jetzt 727); s. XV.
Same as **271** above.
Now *graecus* 271 (coll. 727) (*Census*: 330) nr [1665]).

Dioscurides:
De venenis eorumque praecautione et medicatione.
De iis, quae virus eiaculantur, animalibus libellus, in quo et de rabioso cane.

Venedig, Bibl. Nazionale Marciana, graecus, 272; s. XV.
Now *graecus* 272 (coll. 728) (*Census*: 330, nr [1666]).
See also **272 (jetzt 728)** below.

Dioscurides:
De materia medica (alphab.).

f. 233) *De venenis eorumque praecautione et medicatione.*
(f. 244) *De iis, quae virus eiaculantur, animalibus libellus, in quo et de rabioso cane* (Tit. om.).

Venedig, Bibl. Nazionale Marciana, graecus, 272 (jetzt 728); s. XV.
Same as **272** above.
Now *graecus* 272 (coll. 728) (*Census*: 330, nr [1667]).

Dioscurides:
De venenis eorumque praecautione et medicatione.
De iis, quae virus eiaculantur, animalibus libellus, in quo et de rabioso cane.

Venedig, Bibl. Nazionale Marciana, graecus, 273; s. XII.
Now *graecus* 273 (coll. 669) (*Census*: 330, nr [1668]).

Dioscurides: *De materia medica* (Sine titulo. Ordo et numerus capitum ab editt. discrepat).

Venedig, Bibl. Nazionale Marciana, graecus, 279; s. XV.
Now *graecus* 279 (coll. 705) (*Census*: 330, nr [1674]).

Rufus, Posidonius, Aëtius: *Excerpta varia* (De atra bile, ex libris Galeni, Rufi, Posidonii, Aëtii. »Ex Aetio.« Wellmann).

Venedig, Bibl. Nazionale Marciana, graecus, 281; s. XV.
Now *graecus* 281 (coll. 581) (*Census*: 331, nr [1677]).

Andromachus: (f. 96) *Theriaca.*

Venedig, Bibl. Nazionale Marciana, graecus, 289; s. XV.
Now *graecus* 289 (coll. 627) (*Census*: 332, nr [1687]).

Aëtius Amidenus: *Iatricorum libri XVI* (L. I–VII; »aus derselben Vorlage wie Weigelianus.« M. W.).

Venedig, Bibl. Nazionale Marciana, graecus, 290; s. XV.
Now *graecus* 290 (coll. 628) (*Census*: 332, nr [1688]).

Aëtius Amidenus: *Iatricorum libri XVI* (L. VIII–XVI).

Venedig, Bibl. Nazionale Marciana, graecus, 291; s. XV.
Now *graecus* 291 (coll. 298) (*Census*: 332, nr [1689]).

Aëtius Amidenus: *Iatricorum libri XVI* (»B. I–XVI. Die letzte Seite, fol. 451, stammt aus einer andern Hds. und enthält Bruchstücke des Aëtius, B. VII cap. μζ' · περὶ ἀμβλυωπίας Γαληνοῦ κτλ. Inc. Χιτῶνας καὶ τὸ ὀπτικὸν πνεῦμα. Expl. ὑπαλίφειν ἐλαίῳ παλαιῷ μόνῳ.« M. W.).
Africanus: (f. 499) *De ponderibus et mensuris* (Inc. Ἐπειδὴ πολλαχοῦ σταθμῶν).

Venedig, Bibl. Nazionale Marciana, graecus, 292; a. 1306.
Now *graecus* 292 (coll. 914) (*Census*: 332, nr [1690]).

Paulus Aegineta: (f. 5) *Epitomae medicae libri septem.*

Venedig, Bibl. Nazionale Marciana, graecus, 293; s. XV.
Now *graecus* 293 (coll. 299) (*Census*: 332, nr [1691]).

Paulus Aegineta: (f. 1) *Epitomae medicae libri septem* (*Abschrift von* [Venet. Marcian.] 92 [above p. 168]).
Oribasius: (f. 291) *Excerpta varia* (»Quaedam instar prologi generalis in medicinam quae Oribasio tribuantur«. Inc. *wie im* [Mediol.] Ambros. D 13 Sup. [above p. 74]. Expl. mutil. καὶ ἐὰν διὰ τέλους ...).

Venedig, Bibl. Nazionale Marciana, graecus, 294; s. XIV.
Now *graecus* 294 (coll. 288) (*Census*: 332, nr [1692]).

Oribasius:
Conspectus ad Eustathium filium. Libri II.
(f. 9) *Ad Eunapium de parabilibus medicamentis. Libri IV.*

Venedig, Bibl. Nazionale Marciana, graecus, 295; a. 1470, s. XIV.
s. XIV falso pro a. 1470 [M. W.].
Now *graecus* 295 (coll. 729) (*Census*: 333, nr [1693]).

Alexander Trallianus: (f. 1) *Therapeutica. Libri XII* (Frgm. ex libris XII. *Apographon des* Paris. Suppl. 1297 [above p. 142]).
Paulus Aegineta: (f. 176^{v}) *De mensuris et ponderibus* (Inc. Τὸ ἰταλικὸν κεράμιον. Expl. τὸ μικρὸν μύστρον Γ^{ρ} κ' < ς' < θ'). [M. W.]).
Oribasius: (f. 177^{v}) *Conspectus ad Eustathium filium. Libri IX* (Frgm. »Ohne Überschrift«. Wellmann).
Aelius Promotus: (f. 191^{v}–274^{v}) *Dynameron.*

Venedig, Bibl. Nazionale Marciana, graecus, 296; s. XV.
Now *graecus* 296 (coll. 632) (*Census*: 333, nr [1694]).

Ioannes Zacharias Actuarius: *De urinis libri VII.*

Venedig, Bibl. Nazionale Marciana, graecus, 297; s. XIV.
Now *graecus* 297 (coll. 633) (*Census*: 333, nr [1695]).

Meletius monachus: *De natura hominis.*

Venedig, Bibl. Nazionale Marciana, graecus, 298; s. XV.
Now *graecus* 298 (coll. 583) (*Census*: 333, nr [1696]).

Ioannes Zacharias Actuarius:
De spiritu animali libri II.
De methodo medendi libri VI.

Venedig, Bibl. Nazionale Marciana, graecus, 299; s. XI.
Now *graecus* 299 (coll. 584) (*Census*: 333, nr [1697]).

Stephanus Alexandrinus: *De sacra divinaque arte auri faciendi.*
Democritus: (f. 66^{v}) *Physica et mystica.*
Zosimus Panopolita:
(f. 92) *Liber de virtute et compositione aquarum.*
(f. 113^{v}) *Gemini commentarii de aqua divina* (I).
(f. 115) *Liber de virtute et compositione aquarum.*
(f. 186) *De instrumentis et fornacibus.*
(f. 188) *Gemini commentarii de aqua divina* (II).

Venedig, Bibl. Nazionale Marciana, graecus, 334; s. XIV.
Now *graecus* 334 (coll. 553) (*Census*: 333, nr [1698]).

Hermes Trismegistus: *Methodus ad omne inceptum idonea.*

Venedig, Bibl. Nazionale Marciana, graecus, 335; s. XV.
Now *graecus* 335 (coll. 645) (*Census*: 333, nr [1699]).

Petosiris: *Epistula ad regem Nechepso* (»In indice adnotatur, in codice deest«).
Hermes Trismegistus: (f. 28) *De XII locorum nomenclatura et facultate.*

Venedig, Bibl. Nazionale Marciana, graecus, 336; s. XV, XV–XVI.
Now *graecus* 336 (coll. 646) (*Census*: 333, nr [1700]).

Hermes Trismegistus: *Iatromathematica ad Ammonium Aegyptium.*

Petosiris: (f. 259) *Epistula ad regem Nechepso* (Μέθοδος περὶ νόσων. Inc. *wie im* [Flor.] Laurent. 28, 34 [above p. 41]).

Venedig, Bibl. Nazionale Marciana, graecus, 480; s. –.
Now *graecus* 480 (coll. 589) (*Census*: 333, nr [1701]).

Aglaias: (f. 169) *Ad suffusiones Aglaiae ..., Alexandri discipuli, condiscipuli Demosthenis et amici, versus heroelegi.*

Venedig, Bibl. Nazionale Marciana, graecus, 510; s. XV.
Now *graecus* 510 (coll. 769) (*Census*: 333, nr [1703]).

Ioannes Zacharias Actuarius: *De urinis libri VII* (L. I).

Venedig, Bibl. Nazionale Marciana, graecus, 529; s. XV.
Now *graecus* 529 (coll. 847) (*Census*: 334, nr [1704]).

Ioannes Zacharias Actuarius: *De spiritu animali libri II.*

Venedig, Bibl. Nazionale Marciana, graecus, 596; s. XV.
Now *graecus* 596 (coll. 867) (*Census*: 334, nr [1705]).

Aëtius Amidenus: *Iatricorum libri XVI* (L. I–VIII; «L. I–VIII. Aus ihm stammt die Aldina.» M.W.).

Venedig, Bibl. Nazionale Marciana, graecus, 597; s. XV.
Now *graecus* 597 (coll. 661) (*Census*: 334, nr [1706]).

Dioscurides:
De materia medica (alphab.).
De venenis eorumque praecautione et medicatione.
De iis, quae virus eiaculantur, animalibus libellus, in quo et de rabioso cane.

Venedig, Bibl. Nazionale Marciana, appendix graeca
Now Venezia, Biblioteca Nazionale Marciana, *appendix graeca*

Venedig, Bibl. Nazionale Marciana, appendix graeca, II, 171; s. XV.
Now *app. gr.* II.171 (coll. 445) (*Census*: 334, nr [1708]).

Antyllus: *Excerpta varia* (Ὡς φλεβοτομητέον *und* Περὶ καθάρσεως).
Rufus: *Excerpta varia* (Περὶ ἐμέτων).

Venedig, Bibl. Nazionale Marciana, appendix graeca, IV, 36 (olim Nanian. 258); s. XV–XVI.
Now *app. gr.* IV.36 (coll. 1425) (*Census*: 334, nr [1709]).

Hermes Trismegistus: *Kyranides.*

Venedig, Bibl. Nazionale Marciana, appendix graeca, V, 1; s. XV.
Now *app. gr.* V.1 (coll. 834) (*Census*: 334, nr [1710]).
See also **Padua, Bibl. S. Joannis in Viridario, ad dextr. plut. XVI** above (p. 101).

Paulus Aegineta: *Epitomae medicae libri septem.*

Venedig, Bibl. Nazionale Marciana, appendix graeca, V, 2.
Now *app. gr.* V.2 (coll. 1246) (*Census*: 334, nr [1711]).

Dioscurides: *De materia medica* (Variae lectt. ex duobus codd. mss. manu saec. XVI. in marg. edit. Cornarii Basil. 1529)

Venedig, Bibl. Nazionale Marciana, appendix graeca, V, 3.
Now *app. gr.* V.3 (coll. 1280) (*Census*: 334, nr [1712]).

Dioscurides: *De materia medica* (Edit. Paris. apud Petrum Haultinum a. 1549 cum annotatt. manu Melchioris Guilandini).

Venedig, Bibl. Nazionale Marciana, appendix graeca, V, 8; s. XIV.
Now *app. gr.* V.8 (coll. 1334) (*Census*: 335, nr [1717]).

Beniaminus: (f. 171) *Medicinae variae Beniamini Iudaei* (»Γαλ. καὶ Ἱππ. περὶ βετονίκης in codice legitur; cui opusculo catalogus attribuit titulum Beniamini Iudaei Medicinae variae«).
Taronitus (?): (f. 102v) *Excerpta* (Ἀντίδοτος. λίθος θριπτική).
Ioannes Zacharias Actuarius: (f. 110) *Tractatus de urinis, qui ex Avicenna translatus dicitur in graecam linguam a Christodulo, in ordinem redactus ab Actuario Zacharia.*
Theophilus: (f. 131) *De alvi excrementis* (Expl. καὶ τῶν διὰ μελαγχολικόν).

Venedig, Bibl. Nazionale Marciana, appendix graeca, V, 9; s. XV.
Now *app. gr.* V.9 (coll. 1017) (*Census*: 335, nr [1718]).

Alexander Trallianus:
Therapeutica. Libri XII.
(f. 265–274) *De oculis. Libri III* (L. I et II).

Venedig, Bibl. Nazionale Marciana, appendix graeca, V, 10; s. XVI.
Now *app. gr.* V.10 (coll. 1444) (*Census*: 335, nr [1719]).

Alexander Aphrodisiensis: (f. 1) *Quarundam difficultatum solutiones* (*Wie im* Bonon. [2294] [above p. 24]).

Venedig, Bibl. Nazionale Marciana, appendix graeca, V, 12; s. X–XIII.XV.
Now *app. gr.* V.12 (coll. 1317) (*Census*: 335, nr [1721]).
See also **V, 12 (olim Nanian. 246)** below.

Theophilus:
(f. 98) *De urinis.*
(f. 114) *De alvi excrementis.*
(f. 126) *De pulsibus.*

Venedig, Bibl. Nazionale Marciana, appendix graeca, V, 12 (olim Nanian. 246); s. X–XIII, XV.
Same as **V, 12** above.
Now *app. gr.* V.12 (coll. 1317) (*Census*: 335, nr [1722]).

Theophilus: (f. 39) *De hominis fabrica libri V.*

Venedig, Bibl. Nazionale Marciana, appendix graeca, V, 13; s. XIV–XVI.
Now *app. gr.* V.13 (coll. 1221) (*Census*: 336, nr [1723]).
See also **V, 13 (olim Nanian. 247)** below.

Herophilus Sophista: (f. 1) *De alimentis, quae singulis mensibus sumenda aut vitanda sunt.*
Photius monachus: (f. 5) *Excerpta.*
Methodius Patriarchus: (f. 6) *Excerpta varia* (Inc. Ὁ στόμαχος ἢ κατὰ ποιότητα τρέπει τοὺς σφυγμούς, ἥτις θεωρεῖται. Expl. ὁ ἀνίσως πλήττων τὴν ἁφήν).
Photius monachus: (f. 12) *Excerpta* (Στιχηρὰ ... δοθέντα τῷ εὐσεβεστάτῳ βασιλεῖ κυρίῳ Ἰωάννῃ περὶ μεθόδου ὑαλίων Photii Philosophi. Expl. τῇ δὲ ἕκτῃ ἀπελθέτω εἰς λουτρόν).
Neophytus Prodromenus: (f. 8–25) *Remediorum collectio alphabetica* (Expl. mutil. τῶν ὀλεθρίων ὑφισταμένων τὰ μέν ἐστι κριμνώδη ...).
Ioannes Zacharias Actuarius: (f. 25ᵛ) *De urinis libri VII.*
Paulus Aegineta: (f. 119ᵛ) *Excerpta varia.*
Harpocration: (f. 125) *De facultatibus naturalibus animalium et herbarum et lapidum.*
Aëtius Amidenus: (f. 136) *Excerpta varia* (Π. βοτανῶν κατὰ στοιχεῖον).

Hermes Trismegistus:
(f. 149) *Ad Asclepium de plantis VII planetarum* (Inc. Πρώτη βοτάνη ῞♄ προσαγορευομένη κιχ ρ ῶ).
(f. 157) *De succis plantarum*.

Venedig, Bibl. Nazionale Marciana, appendix graeca, V, 13 (olim Nanian. 247)
Same as **V, 13** above.
Now *app. gr.* V.13 (coll. 1221) (*Census*: 336, nr [1724]).

Hermes Trismegistus: *Kyranides* (L. I. III. II. IV).

Venedig, Bibl. Nazionale Marciana, appendix graeca, V, 15; s. XVI.
Now *app. gr.* V.15 (coll. 1299) (*Census*: 335, nr [1727]).

Erotianus: *Vocum Hippocraticarum conlectio*.

Venedig, Bibl. Nazionale Marciana, appendix graeca, V, 16; s. XVI.
Now *app. gr.* V.16 (coll. 1318) (*Census*: 335, nr [1728]).

Aëtius Amidenus: (f. 42ᵛ) *Excerpta varia* (Π. τροφῶν δυνάμεων Frgm.).
Diocles: (f. 146) *Hippocratis vel, ut alii volunt, Dioclis epistula ad Ptolemaeum Aegypti regem*.
Stephanus Alexandrinus: (f. 148) *In Magni sophistae librum de urinis*.
Dioscurides: (f. 154ᵛ) *Excerpta* (Inc. Μὴν Ἰανουάριος).
Paulus Aegineta: (f. 160ᵛ) *Excerpta varia* (*Wie im* Bonon. 3636. f. 61ᵛ [above p. 26]. Expl. θαυμάσεις πάνυ).
Dioscurides: (f. 161) *Excerpta* (Inc. μελ' τὸ καλόν).
Alexander Aphrodisiensis: (f. 167) *Quarundam difficultatum solutiones* (Ἐπί τισιν ἀπορίαις λύσεις. Inc. Διὰ τί τῶν ἀλόγων ζώων).

Verona

Verona, Bibl. Capitolare, CXXIX (118); s. XVI.

Meletius monachus: (nr 5) *De natura hominis*.

Verona, Bibl. Capitolare, 57 *bei* Montfaucon (*griechisch ?*).
Now Oxford, Bodleian Library, Auct. T. 4. 3 (*Census*: 345, nr [1738]).
Same as **Oxford, Bibl. Bodleiana, Miscell. 241** above (p. 98).

Ioannes Zacharias Actuarius: *Opera*.

Wien

Wien, Vindob. (*bei* Berth.-Ruelle, Alchim. *a. a. O.* [= Alchim. gr. I p. 56–69]).
Possibly Wien, Österreichische Nationalbibliothek, *medicus graecus* 2 (*Census*: 347–348, nr [1741]).

Synesius: *Ad Dioscorum, scholia in librum Democriti.*

Wien, Bibl. Colleg. S. J. Rossianus

Wien, Bibl. Colleg. S. J. Rossianus, XI.167; s. XV.
Now *Vaticanus Rossianus* 982 (*Census*: 348, nr [1742]).

Paulus Nicaeensis: (f. 1) *De cognitione et curatione morborum* (Pinax Inc. α' · περὶ ἐπισκέψεως. Expl. 2^{v} ρλ' · περὶ παρονυχίας).

Paulus Nicaeensis: (f. 12^{v}) *De cognitione et curatione morborum* (de cognitione et curatione variorum morborum. Inc. f. 12^{v} πολλῶν τε καὶ ποικίλων. Expl. f. 135^{v} τὴν σάρκα πανταχόθεν ἀπὸ τοῦ ὄνυχος).

Lucas: (f. 137^{v}) *Compositio salsi intinctus* (Inc. ἔχων ἐνεργείας. Expl. ἐν αὐτῷ τὰς τροφὰς πάσας).

Logadius: (f. 139^{v}) *Excerpta* (σκευασία τῆς ἱερᾶς λογαδίου εἰς ξανθο(χο)λικοὺς καὶ μελαγχολικοὺς καὶ φλεγματικούς. Inc. θύμου οὐγγίαν α'. Expl. 139^{v} ἀφρονίτρου οὐγγίας β').

Rufus: (f. 148^{r}) *Excerpta varia* (σκευασία ἱερᾶς τοῦ ῥούφου τοῦ ἐφεσίου εἰς δυσπνοιικοὺς καὶ δυσουριῶντας καὶ παχυφλεγματικούς. Inc. Χαμανδρίνου οὐγγίας ι'. Expl. μέλιτος ἀπηφρισμένον τὸ ἀρκοῦν).

Syncellus: (f. 153^{v}) *Excerpta* (σκευασία συγκέλλου τοῦ πανολβίου. Inc. πεπέρεως κοινοῦ. Expl. μέλιτος τὸ ἀρκοῦν).

Esdras Propheta: (f. 156) *Pro hydropicis et omnibus morbis frigidis* (Inscr. καὶ ἡ τρίτη σκευασία τοῦ ἔσδρακος τοῦ σοφοῦ καὶ μεγάλου προφήτου εἰς – νοσήματα. Inc. μαμηρά, οὐγγίαν ᾱ. Expl. ἀπηφρισμένον τὸ ἀρκοῦν).

Philo: (f. 156^{r}) *Excerpta varia* (Φίλωνος · φιλῶ τὴν σκευασίαν πάνυ εἰς φλεγματικοὺς καὶ πνευματικούς. Inc. κρόκου οὐγγίας β'. Expl. καὶ μέλιτος τὸ ἀρκοῦν).

Wien, Hofbibliothek, Vindob./Vindobon.
Now Wien, Österreichische Nationalbibliothek, *Vindobonenses*

Wien, Hofbibliothek, hist. 94; x. XVI.

Asclepiades: (f. 61v) *Praecepta salubria* (Sine auctoris nomine. Expl. σύκοις δὲ συχνοῖς καὶ σταφυλαῖς ἐκτρέφου).

Wien, Hofbibliothek, Vindob. lat. 16 (Tab. cod. I p. 2 s.); s. VIII–IX.

Dioscurides: (f. 62, 65 rescr.) *De materia medica* (Lib. III 82. 83. 78. 79 ed. Wellm.).

Wien, Hofbibliothek, Vindob. med. 1; s. V–VI, VI in., VI.

Dioscurides: (f. 12v) *De materia medica* (Inscr. *wie im* Phillipps. Cheltenham 3084 [above p. 30]. Inc. Ἀείζων τὸ μέγα. Expl. *wie im* [Cheltenham] Phil. 3084).
Crateuas: (f. 18v) *De herbis* (Frgm.).
Eutecnius:
(f. 393–437v) *Paraphrasis in Nicandri Theriaca.*
(f. 438v) *Paraphrasis in Nicandri Alexipharmaca.*
(f. 460) *Paraphrasis in Oppiani Halieutica* (Inscriptionis expers).
(f. 474–485v) *Paraphrasis in Dionysii Ixeutica* (Inc. ...ψιεις, εἰ καὶ πόρρω που τελευτήσεις, τι τῶν ζώων. Expl. Ἀπόλλωνος δὲ μ̣α̣λ̣χ̣ε̣α̣ι̣).

Wien, Hofbibliothek, Vindob. med. 3; s. –.

Ioannes Zacharias Actuarius: (f. 136–230) *De urinis libri VII.*

Wien, Hofbibliothek, Vindob. med. 5; s. XVI, XVI–XVII.

Crateuas: *De herbis* (»E Vindob. med. 1.« Wellmann).
Eutecnius: (f. 9) *Paraphrasis in Nicandri Alexipharmaca* (Frgm. Inc. Νίκανδρος ὁ ποιητής. Expl. πρὸς σωτηρίαν τῶν ἀνθρώπων καὶ ὠφέλειαν ἐξεύρηται. *Aus* Vindob. med. 1 [above]).

Wien, Hofbibliothek, Vindob. med. 6; s. –.

Crateuas: *De herbis* (Frgm.).
Aëtius Amidenus: (f. 3) *Iatricorum libri XVI* (Expl. καὶ ὠφελεῖ τοὺς ἐμέτους. *Coll. mit der Ald. von Weigel im Berol. fol. 39 [275]* [above p. 15]).

Wien, Hofbibliothek, Vindob. med. 8; s. XV.

Meletius monachus: (f. 1) *De natura hominis* (Τὰ περὶ τῆς τοῦ ἀνθρώπου κατασκευῆς. Expl. καὶ αἰσχυνομένης ἐρυθρὸν σῶμα δείκνυται).
Theophilus: (f. 57ᵛ) *De alvi excrementis.*
Paulus Aegineta:
(f. 64) *Epitomae medicae libri septem* (L. I–VI χειρισμόν; *vgl.* Parisin. 2191 [above p. 118]).
(f. 240) *De succedaneis, ex Galeno.*
Antyllus: (f. 278ᵛ) *Excerpta varia* (*Wie im* [Rom] Barberin. [I 127] [above p. 146]).
Paulus Aegineta: (f. 281ᵛ) *De mensuris et ponderibus* (Expl. wie im [Lond. Brit. Mus.] Harleian [6305] [above p. 65]).
Rufus: (f. 283) *Quaestiones medicinales.*
Petosiris: (f. 294) *Epistula ad regem Nechepso* (*Wie im* Cracov. [2526] [above p. 57]).
Ioannes Episcopus Prisdianensis: (f. 320) *Collectanea de urinis.*
Theophilus: (f. 320ᵛ) *De urinis.*

Wien, Hofbibliothek, Vindob. med. 10; s. XVI.

Alexander Aphrodisiensis: (f. 1) *De febribus.*

Wien, Hofbibliothek, Vindob. med. 11; s. –.

Dioscurides: *Liber agens de experientia medica, de simplicibus et compositis medicamentis, ordine literarum digestus.*
Diocles: (f. 56) *Ad Antigonum regem epistula de tuenda valetitudine* (Expl. ἐστὶ τὸ ὠάλοιμα ὠφελοῦν εἰς καψίδα ὀφθαλμῶν).

Wien, Hofbibliothek, Vindob. med. 12; s. XV.
s. XIV–XV.

Aëtius Amidenus: (f. 1–269ᵛ) *Iatricorum libri XVI* (Expl. τεθαμβημέναν ὄκνον πρὸς ...; L. IX init. mut. *Apogr. des Parisin.* 2191 [above p. 118]).
Paulus Aegineta: (f. 92–142) *Epitomae medicae libri septem* (Liber VI).

Wien, Hofbibliothek, Vindob. med. 14; s. –, XVI.

Dioscurides: (f. 1–46ᵛ) *De materia medica* (Sine titulo. Lib. I *und* II 1–26. Expl. δριμὺ δηκτικὸν εὔτριπτον δια ...).

Wien, Hofbibliothek, Vindob. med. 15; s. –.
s. XV.
See (possibly) **[15]** below.

Marcellinus: (f. 101) *De pulsibus.*

[Wien, Hofbibliothek, Vindob. med. 15].
Possibly same as **Wien, Hofbibliothek, Vindob. med. 15** above (*Census*: 358, nr [1779]).
= ? *medicus graecus* 15.

Alexander Aphrodisiensis: *De febribus.*

Wien, Hofbibliothek, Vindob. med. 16; s. XV–XVI.
s. XV.
See also **med. 16 (ol. 35)** below.

Stephanus Atheniensis: *De febrium differentiis ex ore Theophili* (Sine auctoris nomine. Περιτομὴ τοῦ περὶ διαφορᾶς πυρετῶν).
Theophilus: *Commentarius in Hippocratis aphorismos* (Expl. δηλοῖ γὰρ ἐπίτασιν ξηρότητος. *Abschrift im Berol. fol. 39 [275]* [above p. 15]).
Dioscurides:
(f. 43–48ᵛ, 56) *De materia medica* (»Fragmentum D. alphab.« M. Wellmann).
(f. 56) *De materia medica* (Frgm. »D. libris V digestus«. M. Wellmann. Expl. f. 184ᵛ ἐπ' ὠφελείᾳ διδομένω [sic] ἕνεκα τῶν ἐπιφερομένων κινδύνων).
Stephanus Atheniensis: (f. 185) *In aphorismos Hippocratis commentarius* (Sine auctoris nomine. Σχόλια εἰς τοὺς Ἱππ. ἀφορ. κατὰ σύνοψιν. Inc. Ὅρος ἀφορισμοῦ. Ἀφορισμός ἐστι λόγος σύντομος. Expl. δηλοῖ γὰρ ἐπίτασιν ξηρότητος).
Marcellinus: (f. 319) *De pulsibus* (Μαρκέλλου περὶ σφυγμῶν. Inc. Σφυγμῶν θι..ειν καὶ σφυγμῶν ὅσα χρὴ μαθεῖν. Expl. παλαιας εἰς εὕρεσιν διδούς).
Theophilus: (f. 325ᵛ–328ᵛ) *Epitome librorum Galeni de febrium differentiis.*

Wien, Hofbibliothek, Vindob. med. 16 (ol. 35); s. –, XV.
Same as **16** above (*Census*: 358–359, nr [1781]).
= *medicus graecus* 16.

Oribasius: *Medicae collectiones ad Iulianum* (Capp. 43 extr. 44 librorum incert. = Oribas. III p. 230 sq. Dbg.-Buss.).

Wien, Hofbibliothek, Vindob. med. 18; s. –, XV, XVI.

Stephanus Atheniensis: *Dioscoridis et Stephani Atheniensis de pharmacis ordine literarum* (»Proben« *im Berol. fol. 39 [275]* [above p. 15]).
Dioscurides: (f. 94) *Liber agens de experientia medica, de simplicibus et compositis medicamentis, ordine literarum digestus* (*Wie im* cod. bibl. Io. Rhodii [above p. 100]).

Wien, Hofbibliothek, Vindob. med. 21; s. –.

Ioannes Zacharias Actuarius:
(f. 1–119) *De urinis libri VII.*
(f. 120–173) *De spiritu animali libri II.*
(f. 173–267ᵛ) *De methodo medendi libri VI* (L. I–III).
(f. 268–303) *De methodo medendi libri VI* (L. VI cap. 1–31).
Paulus Aegineta: (f. 303–306) *De succedaneis, ex Galeno.*
Ioannes Zacharias Actuarius: (f. 307–415ᵛ) *De methodo medendi libri VI* (L. IV–V).

Wien, Hofbibliothek, Vindob. med. 22; s. –, XV.

Ioannes Zacharias Actuarius: (f. 1–55) *De methodo medendi libri VI* (L. IV. V).
Diocles: (f. 56–60) *Ad Antigonum regem epistula de tuenda valetitudine.*

Wien, Hofbibliothek, Vindob. med. 23; s. –, XVI.

Ioannes Zacharias Actuarius: (f. 1) *De methodo medendi libri VI* (Libri VI sub nomime Pyropuli [?]).
Hermes Trismegistus:
(f. 1–76) *De succis plantarum* (Βίβλοι ἰατρικαὶ σύντομοι κατὰ μαθηματικῆς ἐπιστήμης ... ἐκδοθεῖσαι πρὸς μαθητὴν αὐτοῦ Ἀσκληπιόν, περὶ ἄστρων, βοτανῶν, τῶν ζώων, τῶν πηγῶν, τῶν τετραπόδων, τῶν ἐναλίων ἰχθύων τε καὶ ναυτῶν, τῶν ἄστρων τε καὶ λίθων δυνάμεως. Inc. f. 1 Κριοῦ ἐλελίσφακος. Expl. f. 76 ὡς ἔγωγε πεπείρακα).
(f. 18) *De decanis ad Asclepium* (Inc. Τῶν ἐν τοῖς ζωδίοις τριακονταὲξ δεκανῶν. Expl. ἰδίαν γὰρ δύναμιν φυσικῶς ἔλαβεν βοτάνη).
(f. 76) *De ponderibus* (Περὶ τῶν δηλούντων τοὺς σταθμοὺς διὰ τῶν χαρακτήρων. Inc. Ὁ μακάριος τρισκαταιόφρων Ἑρμῆς. Expl. ἔτι δὲ καὶ οὕτως θ'' τὸ ἔνατον).
Paulus Aegineta: (f. 76) *De mensuris et ponderibus* (Frgm. Inscr. Ἑρμοῦ τοῦ τρισμεγίστου. Inc. Ὁ μακάριος τρισκραταιόφρων Ἐρμῆς. Expl. καὶ οὕτως θ'' τὸ ἔννατον).

Hermes Trismegistus: *Excerpta varia*:

(f. 77ᵛ) Περὶ τῶν μελῶν τοῦ ἀνθρώπου, ὅταν λαγγέβουν, γνώριζε οὕτως. Inc. Ὀφρὺς δεξιὸς ἐὰν ἅλυται [sic] ἐν ὀλίγῳ χρόνῳ. Expl. πολλῶν ἀγαθῶν ἐπιτυχίαν δηλοῖ.

(f. 79ᵛ) Περὶ τῶν φριλτῶν [sic !], ὅπως τὸ ἕνα ὑπόκειται ὑπὸ τῆς δεκάδος καὶ ἡ δεκὰς ὑπὸ τῆς ἑκατοντάδος. Inc. [Kryptogr.] σεῆηνσωπεϛνωε. Expl. σλω · πθσ'λ̆ψ.

Wien, Hofbibliothek, Vindob. med. 25; s. XV, XV–XVI.

Paulus Aegineta: (f. 10) *De mensuris et ponderibus* (Frgm. Περὶ τῶν δηλούντων τοὺς σταθμοὺς καὶ τὰ μέτρα χαρακτήρων. Inc. Ἀλλ' ἐπειδή τινες. Expl. *wie im* [Lond. Brit. Mus.] Harleian. [6305] [above p. 65]).

Wien, Hofbibliothek, Vindob. med. 26; s. XV.

Ioannes Zacharias Actuarius:

(f. 1) *De urinis libri VII* (Ὀκταρίου).

(f. 244–303) *De methodo medendi libri VI* (L. III. VI).

Paulus Aegineta: (f. 303–305ᵛ) *De succedaneis, ex Galeno* (Expl. ἀντὶ ὠκίμου σισύμβριον).

Ioannes Zacharias Actuarius: (f. 307–412) *De methodo medendi libri VI* (Inc. *wie im* Londin. Medical Society NNa 11 = Wf 8 [above p. 67]).

Wien, Hofbibliothek, Vindob. med. 27; s. XVI.

Diocles: (f. 101) *Ad Antigonum regem epistula de tuenda valetitudine.*

Hermes Trismegistus: (f. 104ᵛ) *De ponderibus* (Περὶ σταθμῶν. Inc. Ὁ σταθμὸς βάρει μετρούμενος κρίνεται. Expl. μάλιστα συνήθων ἡμῖν ὁ λόγος).

Paulus Aegineta: (f. 104ᵛ) *De mensuris et ponderibus* (Frgm. Inc. Ἀλλὰ διὰ τῶν χαρακτήρων ταῦτα. Expl. *wie im* Vindob. med. 23 [above p. 181]).

Severianus: (f. 113ᵛ–114) *De hominis nomine.*

Epiphanius: (f. 118ᵛ–121) *De duodecim gemmis panno sacerdotis infibulatis.*

Esdras Propheta: (f. 121) *De diebus criticis* (Περὶ τῶν δώδεκα μηνῶν τὰς ἐπιβαρεῖς ἡμέρας. Inc. Μηνὶ σεπτεβρίῳ γ'. Expl. Αὔγουστος δ' καὶ ιε').

Oribasius: (f. 122) *Excerpta varia* (Περὶ τὸ πῶς χρὴ γιγνώσκειν τὸ αἷμα. Inc. Δεῖ σε γινώσκειν τοῦτο ὅτι τὸ αἷμα ὃ προφαίνεται. Expl. ἵνα μὴ διαβοῦν καὶ τὰ ἔγκατα αὐτῆς).

Wien, Hofbibliothek, Vindob. med. 28; s. –, XV.

Dioscurides: *Liber agens de experientia medica, de simplicibus et compositis medicamentis, ordine literarum digestus.*

Herophilus Sophista: *De alimentorum facultatibus.*

Theophilus:

(f. 2) *Excerpta varia* (Ab init. mutil. Inc. Οἱ δὲ πελιοί. Expl. τὰ δὲ ἄλλα φυλάττουσιν κατὰ φ... + τέλος σὺν θεῷ ἁγίῳ τὸ περὶ σφυγμῶν ἀπὸ φωνῆς Θεοφίλου ἐκ τοῦ προγνωστικοῦ Γαληνοῦ).

(f. 18) *Epitome librorum Galeni de febrium differentiis* (Πόσαι διαφοραὶ πυρετῶν. Inc. Διαφοραὶ τῶν πυρετῶν αἱ μὲν οἰκειόταται. Expl. f. 26ᵛ καὶ ἐκφεύξῃ θάνατον ἐκ κερασμάτων [?]).

Dioscurides: (f. 67–115) *De materia medica – Excerpta* (Inscr. Βίβλος ἑρμηνεὺς πόων βοτανῶν κτλ. κατὰ στοιχεῖον. Inc. Ἀψίνθιον. Expl. ὤκιμον).

Aëtius Amidenus: (f. 118–139ᵛ) *Iatricorum libri XVI* (Exc. l. II 3. 75 etc.).

Lucas: (f. 156) *Compositio salsi intinctus* (Inc. Ὀφθαλμῶν οὗ πιεῖ. Expl. ἀνὰ κοχλιαρίων δυοῖν ἢ καὶ τριῶν).

Meletius monachus: (f. 164–183) *De natura hominis* (Frgm. Ἐπιτομὴ π. τῆς κατασκευῆς τοῦ ἀνθρώπου κτλ. Inc. *wie im* Scorial. [y. I. 15] [above p. 36]. Expl. ἐν κόπρῳ ἐν οὔρῳ ἐν πτίσμασι ...).

Paulus Aegineta: (f. 186ᵛ. 187ᵛ) *Excerpta varia* (Π. φλεβοτομίας. Inc. *wie im* [Vatic.] Palat. 279. f. 212ᵛ [above p. 150]. Expl. καὶ τῶν ἀλλοτρίων ἀποκριτικήν).

Wien, Hofbibliothek, Vindob. med. 29; s. XV.

Theophilus: (f. 1–8ᵛ) *De urinis* (Frgm. Inc. Ἐρώτησις πῶς γίνεται. Expl. ἐγκυμονούσης ἐστίν).

Paulus Aegineta: (f. 12–22ᵛ) *Excerpta varia* (Inc. *wie im* [Vatic.] Palat. 279. f. 212ᵛ [above p. 150]. Expl. τὸν καθαρισμὸν τοῦ ἐγκεφάλου ἐξάγον).

Dioscurides: (f. 22ᵛ–73) *De materia medica* (*Wie in* [Vindob. med.] *nr.* 28 [above]. Expl. ἐν τῷ ὑπογαίῳ ἀποθνήσκει).

Epiphanius:

(f. 117) *Physiologus* (Inc. Ἀρξώμεθα τοίνυν λαλῆσαι περὶ τοῦ λέοντος βασιλέως. Expl. θηρεύονται παρὰ τοῦ θηρευτεοῦ).

(f. 464ᵛ–475) *De duodecim gemmis panno sacerdotis infibulatis* (Expl. τίθει δὲ ἐντὸς τῶν ὀφθαλμῶν περισσότερον).

Paulus Aegineta: (f. 459ᵛ) *De succedaneis, ex Galeno.*

Wien, Hofbibliothek, Vindob. med. 31; s. –, XV ex.

s. XV.

Paulus Nicaeensis: (f. 1–126ᵛ) *De cognitione et curatione variorum morborum.*

Esdras Propheta: (f. 127 [hinter]) *Pro hydropicis et omnibus morbis frigidis.*

Lucas: (f. 127 [hinter]; 130ᵛ–131) *Compositio salsi intinctus.*

Esdras Propheta: (f. 133–133ᵛ) *Pro hydropicis et omnibus morbis frigidis.*

Logadius: (f. 133v–136v) *Excerpta.*
Rufus: (f. 150r–150v) *Excerpta varia.*
Syncellus: (f. 159r–159v) *Excerpta.*
Philo: (f. 163) *Excerpta varia.*
Nicomedes: (f. 166v) *Versus in Hippocratem.*

Wien, Hofbibliothek, Vindob. med. 32; s. XVI.

Dioscurides: (f. 29–30v) *Liber agens de experientia medica, de simplicibus et compositis medicamentis, ordine literarum digestus* (Expl. ὁ τοιοῦτος ἀνέλπιστος).
Paulus Aegineta: (f. 31) *De mensuris et ponderibus* (Frgm. Inc. Τὸ ἡμίεκτον. Expl. ἑρμηνία τῶν σταθμῶν καὶ μέτρων καὶ ⟨π⟩ερὶ ἐλαίου καὶ οἴνου ... ἐτελειώθησαν)
Diocles: (f. 111v) *Ad Antigonum regem epistula de tuenda valetitudine* (Expl. περὶ τῶν ἅπασι μάλιστα συνήθων ἡμῶν ὁ λόγος).

Wien, Hofbibliothek, Vindob. med. 37; s. –, XV.

Herodotus: (f. 13–38v) *Diagnostica de morbis acutis et chronicis* (Inc. φάσκων = Parisin. Suppl. 636. f. 49, 8. Expl. καὶ τὸ διὰ τοῦ μυρο| ... = Paris. Suppl. 636. f. 82, 16 [above p. 140]).
Theophilus: (f. 75v) *De alvi excrementis* (»Ein Blatt«).

Wien, Hofbibliothek, Vindob. med. 38 c; s. –.

Erotianus: *Vocum Hippocraticarum conlectio.*

Wien, Hofbibliothek, Vindob. med. 39; s. –, a. 1561.

Dioscurides: *Liber agens de experientia medica, de simplicibus et compositis medicamentis, ordine literarum digestus.*
Muscio: (f. 5v–52v) *De morbis mulierum* (Inc. Ὁπηνίκα συνεχῶς ἡμῖν ἐν ταῖς γυναιξὶν ἡ μαῖα ἐγεγόνει. Expl. ἢ φόβου ἢ ὀργιλότητος).

Wien, Hofbibliothek, Vindob. med. 40; s. XV.

Paulus Aegineta: (f. 65–71) *De succedaneis, ex Galeno* (Expl. *wie im* Vindob. [med. gr.] 26 [above p. 182]).

Wien, Hofbibliothek, Vindob. med. 41; s. XIV.
s. XIV–XV.

Paulus Nicaeensis: (f. 1) *De cognitione et curatione variorum morborum* (Inc. mutil. cap. ιη' med. διακρατήσω οὖν καὶ μαλακῶς τρίψας).
Lucas: (f. 88–89) *Compositio salsi intinctus.*

Esdras Propheta: (f. 92ᵛ–93ᵛ) *Pro hydropicis et omnibus morbis frigidis.*
Logadius: (f. 93ᵛ–96) *Excerpta.*
Rufus: (f. 115v–116ᵛ) *Excerpta varia.*
Syncellus: (f. 127–127ᵛ) *Excerpta.*
Philo: (f. 132) *De pulsibus.*

Wien, Hofbibliothek, Vindob. med. 42; s. XVI–XVII.

Oribasius: (f. 1–333) *Conspectus ad Eustathium filium. Libri II* (Expl. βέβαιον λάβωμεν περὶ τοῦ μένειν κατεσταλμένον. »Die letzten Capitel des I. Buches, von Buch IV das Cap. de aquis u. die Bücher V–XI [*IX?*]. «).

Wien, Hofbibliothek, Vindob. med. 43; s. XVI.

Erotianus: (f. 83–121ᵛ) *Vocum Hippocraticarum conlectio.*
Soranus: (f. 122) *Hippocratis genus et vita secundum Soranum* (Inc. Πρῶτον τὴν ἐπωνυμίαν. Expl. ἐν περιόδοισιν ὅτι ἑβδομήκοντα κινέεται. »Wahrscheinlich nicht hierhergehörig.« Schoene).

Wien, Hofbibliothek, Vindob. med. 44; s. XV.XVI, XV–XVI.

Stephanus Atheniensis: (f. 1) *In aphorismos Hippocratis commentarius* (Inc. ἐν τῇσι = Dietz p. 283, 3).
Theophilus: (f. 1–126ᵛ) *Commentarius in Hippocratis aphorismos* (*Vgl.* Stephanus).
Stephanus Atheniensis: (f. 127–135ᵛ) *De febrium differentiis ex ore Theophili* (Expl. τοῦ ἐπὶ ζέσει τοῦ αἵματος γινομένου πυρετοῦ).
Ioannes Zacharias Actuarius: (f. 136) *De urinis libri VII.*
Alexander Aphrodisiensis: (f. 231) *Quarundam difficultatum solutiones* (Inc. *wie im* [Venet.] Marc. App. V 16 [above p. 176]. Expl. καὶ βλέφαρα οἰδαλέα καὶ ἀπλότριχα καὶ πολιώδη).

Wien, Hofbibliothek, Vindob. med. 45; s. XV.

Meletius monachus: (f. 1–27) *De natura hominis* (Inc. *wie im* Scorial. [y. I. 15] [above p. 36]).

Wien, Hofbibliothek, Vindob. med. 48; s. XIV–XV.

Romanus: (f. 1–46) *De morbis acutis et chronicis* (Inscr. Ῥωμανοῦ κουβουκλισίου κτλ. Expl. κἂν συνάγῃ στύφοντα κἂν σκληρύνῃ μαλάγματα).
Paulus Aegineta: (f. 197–236ᵛ) *Epitomae medicae libri septem* (L. I–III in. Expl. διὰ τῆς ἱερᾶς ἀντιδότου καθαίρωμεν φλέγματός τε ...).

Wien, Hofbibliothek, Vindob. med. 49; s. XVI.

Ptolemaeus: (f. 22–30v) *Excerpta varia* (Καρπός. Προεκθέμενοι, ὦ Σύρε. Expl. ἐγχώριος ἔσται ὁ ἐχθρός).

Wien, Hofbibliothek, Vindob. med. 50; s. –.

Hermes Trismegistus: *Kyranides*.

Wien, Hofbibliothek, Vindob. med. 51; s. –.

Aëtius Amidenus: *Iatricorum libri XVI* (*L. VIII coll. von Weigel im Berol. 39 [275]* [above p. 15]).

Wien, Hofbibliothek, Vindob. med. 52; s. –, XV.

Aëtius Amidenus: *Iatricorum libri XVI*.
Theophilus: (f. 1–22v) *Epitome librorum Galeni de febrium diferentiis* (Θεόφ. καὶ Στέφ. ἔκ τε Ἱππ. καὶ Γαλ. π. τῆς τ. πυρ. διαφ. Expl. θερμασίας αὗται γίνονται).
Dioscurides: (f. 39–48) *Liber agens de experientia medica, de simplicibus et compositis medicamentis, ordine literarum digestus* (Expl. καὶ διακρατούμενον).
Herophilus Sophista: (f. 60–66v) *De alimentorum facultatibus* (Expl. mutil. φακῇ καὶ κράμβη διὰ τοῦτο καὶ τὴν ὄψιν ἀμβλύνουσι, πλὴν εἰ τύχοι ὑγρότερος ...).

Wien, Hofbibliothek, Vindob. med. 53; s. XVI.

Meletius monachus: (f. 129–189) *Excerpta varia* (Ἰατροσόφιον. Capita 112. Inc. Περὶ ἐντέρων ὅταν ἐξέβουν. Expl. διὰ τί ἔνε καλὸς καιρός).

Wien, Hofbibliothek, Vindob. phil. 34; s. XVI.
Now *philos. et philol. gr.* 34 (*Census*: 362: nr [1818]).

Nemesius Emesenus: *De natura hominis* (*aus Dresd. Da 57* [above p. 32]).

Wien, Hofbibliothek, Vindob. phil. 37; s. XV–XVI.
Now *philos. et philol. gr.* 37 (*Census*: 362: nr [1819]).

Petosiris: *Epistula ad regem Nechepso* (cap. ρκη').

Wien, Hofbibliothek, Vindob. phil. 74; s. XVI.
Now *philos. et philol. gr.* 74 (*Census*: 362: nr [1820]).

Theophilus: (f. 52–107v) *Commentarius in Hippocratis aphorismos* (Expl. πάντως ἂν εἴη ἴαμα. *Vgl.* Oxford [Bodl.] Roe 14 [above p. 99]).

Wien, Hofbibliothek, Vindob. phil. 108; s. XVI.
Now *philos. et philol. gr.* 108 (*Census*: 362: nr [1822]).

Petosiris:
(f. 162) *Organum de vita et morte* (Περὶ Πετ. ὄργανον πρὸς Νεχεψὼ τῷ βασιλεῖ. *Vgl. die* Ἐπιστολὴ πρὸς Νεχ.).
(f. 232) *Excerpta* (Περὶ συμφώνων τῶν τετραγώνων θαυμάσιον. Inc. Ὑπολαμβάνουσι πάντες. Expl. τὸ πράσσειν ἔχοντες ἐστηριγμένοι. Ed. *im* Catal. cod. astrol. gr. VI p. 62).

Wien, Hofbibliothek, Vindob. phil. 178; s. XV.
Now *philos. et philol. gr.* 178 (*Census*: 362: nr [1823]).

Paulus Aegineta: (f. 24v–25v) *De mensuris et ponderibus* (Inc. Ὁ σταθμός. Expl. μικρὸν μύστρον <θ).
Asclepiades: (f. 35) *Praecepta salubria* (Ὑγ. π. σύντομα Ἀσκλ. ταῦτα καὶ Διοσκορίδους).
Theophylactus Simocatta: (f. 305v) *Quaestiones naturales* (Anonym; Ideler p. 174, 13 – 183, 22).

Wien, Hofbibliothek, Vindob. phil. 181; s. XVII.
Now *philos. et philol. gr.* 181 (*Census*: 362: nr [1825]).

Nemesius Emesenus: (f. 171) *De natura hominis* (Frgm. ἀδαμαντίνου νεμεσίνου [!]; *capp. 9–11. 16 Schl. 18–44 fehlen*).

Wien, Hofbibliothek, Vindob. phil. 290; s. –.
Now *philos. et philol. gr.* 290 (*Census*: 362: nr [1828]).

Epiphanius: *Physiologus.*

Wien, Hofbibliothek, Vindob. phil. 303; s. XVI.
Now *philos. et philol. gr.* 303 (*Census*: 362: nr [1829]).

Rufus: (f. 1–16v) *De corporis humani appellationibus.*

Wien, Hofbibliothek, Vindob. suppl. 8; s. XVII.

Aëtius Amidenus: *Iatricorum libri XVI* (L. VIII–XVI. Inc. Προείρηται μὲν περὶ τούτου).

Wien, Hofbibliothek, Vindob. suppl. 28 (olim Neapolitan.); s. VII.
Now Naples, Biblioteca Nazionale Vittorio Emanuele III, *Neapolitanus olim vindobonensis graecus* I (*Census*: 365, nr [1832]).

Dioscurides: (f. 1–172) *De materia medica* (Inc. Ἀριστολοχία μακρά. Expl. Χαμαικίσσου ... ἑπτὰ ἡμέρας).

Wien, Hofbibliothek, Vindob. suppl. 81; s. XVI.

Aëtius Amidenus: (f. 1–307ᵛ) *Iatricorum libri XVI* (L. VIII–XIII. Inc. Ἀσκληπιάδου τροχίσκος. Expl. ἐκ προδήλου αἰτίας).

Wien, Hofbibliothek, Vindob. theol. 68; s. XVI.

Nemesius Emesenus: *De natura hominis* (*aus Monac. 419 abgeschr.* [above p. 88]).

Wien, Hofbibliothek, Vindob. theol. 128; s. –.

Epiphanius: *Physiologus.*

Wien, Hofbibliothek, Vindob. theol. 199; s. XVI.

Nemesius Emesenus: (f. 1) *De natura hominis* (Frgm.).

Wien, Hofbibliothek, Vindob. theol. 207; s. –.
= ? *theologicus graecus* 315 (*Census*: 367, nr [1837]).

Splenius philosophus: (f. 61ᵛ) *De generatione hominis* (Sub nomine Splenii).

Wolfenbüttel, Bibl. Guelf. August.
Now Wolfenbüttel, Herzog August Bibliothek Wolfenbüttel

Wolfenbüttel, Bibl. Guelf. August., Guelferbyt. Ebert. 2 (47 Gud. gr.); s. –.
= 47 Gud. graec. fol. (*Census*: 369, nr [1842]).
See also **Guelferbyt. 2 (Gud. 47)** below.

Paulus Aegineta: *Epitomae medicae libri septem.*

Wolfenbüttel, Bibl. Guelf. August., Guelferbyt. 2 (Gud. 47); s. –.
= 47 Gud. graec. fol. (*Census*: 369, nr [1843]).
See also **Guelferbyt. Ebert. 2 (47 Gud. gr.)** above.

Paulus Aegineta: *Epitomae medicae libri septem.*

Zaragoza

Zaragoza, Bibl. d. Cat. d. Pil., 1106 (ol. 562); s. XV.
Now New Haven, Yale University, Harvey Cushing/John Hay Whitney Medical Library, Manuscript 32 vault (*Census*: 372, nr [1855]).

Rufus:
(f. 2) *Nomenclatura rerum ad hominem pertinentium. Libri III.*
(f. 6ᵛ) *De dissectione partium corporis humani.*
(f. 16) *De ossibus.*

Zaragoza, Bibl. d. Cat. d. Pil., 1115 (olim 1427); s. XVI.
Now New Haven, Yale University, Harvey Cushing/John Hay Whitney Medical Library, Manuscript 50 vault (*Census*: 372–373, nr [1856]).

Damascius: (f. 1) *Expositio in Prognostica Hippocratis. Sectiones II.*

Zürich, Stadtbibliothek
Now Zürich, Zentralbibliothek Zürich – Kantons-, Stadt- und Universitätsbibliothek

Zürich, Stadtbibliothek, Turicens. C 50; s. XVI.
Now MS. C 50 (*Census*: 373, nr [1858]).

Stephanus Atheniensis: (f. 1) *Dioscoridis et Stephani Atheniensis de pharmacis ordine literarum.*

Zürich, Stadtbibliothek, C 136; s. XVI.
Now MS. C 136 (*Census*: 373, nr [1859]).

Dioscurides: *Excerpta*:
(f. 115) περὶ τοῦ οἴνου.
(f. 120) περὶ λυκίου, μυρίκης, σπληνός, λέπρας.

www.ingramcontent.com/pod-product-compliance
Ingram Content Group UK Ltd.
Pitfield, Milton Keynes, MK11 3LW, UK
UKHW050953290926
15470UKWH00006B/1804

9 783110 600698